Tracie O'Keefe
Katrina Fox
Editors

Trans People in Love

Pre-publication
REVIEWS,
COMMENTARIES,
EVALUATIONS . . .

"**P**erfect for anyone interested in exploring the often treacherous waters of love and relationships. The magic of this book is that each love story has elements all people can relate to, regardless of gender or sexuality. A touching demonstration of how love has the power to transcend adversity, sometimes, except when it falls flat on it's face. A warts-and-all collection of first-person narratives that give space and form to all trans people who have previously and historically been forced to deny sexual and romantic relationships. . . . Compelling in freshness . . . emphasis on content over literary style. Like an avocado, you won't know what you're getting until you open it."

Del LaGrace Volcano
Author, *The Drag King Book with Judith Halberstam* and *Femmes of Power: Exploding Queer Femininities with Ulrika Dahl*

"**S**tories like these have probably been sought but never before found in such a large collection. . . . For those who need proof and affirmations on positive human capacities, this book renders insights that human beings can move way beyond what is commonly perceived as sex and gender, and still they stay within the endless capacities of love."

Esben Esther Pirelli Benestad
Physician, Associate Professor, University of Agder, Specialist in Clinical Sexology NACS, Family Therapist IAP

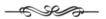

"**D**o not neglect this book as just another [one] on transexuality or transgender. . . . It is written sympathetically and will temper insight for professional readers of different disciplines and those in Gender Studies. Transpeople will be able to view lifestyles of others. Social commentators will be attracted."

Professor A W Steinbeck, MB,BS,MD (Syd), Phd (Lond), FRCP (Lond), FRACP previously of Faculty of Medicine, University of New South Wales, Sydney; Endocrine Society, USA and Australia

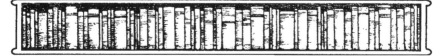

More pre-publication
REVIEWS, COMMENTARIES, EVALUATIONS . . .

"Dip into this book at random, as you can be confident that each chapter is uniformly delightful but different. Each contributor's experience of love and relationships is intricately bound to their uniquely nuanced understanding of what their gender means to them. If you take gender for granted then the tableau for viewing relationships is limited to that common conception. Yet each of these articulate souls shows that a richer and personalized vocabulary of gender leads to many more possibilities for love too. The genius of the editors is in capturing these different visions."

Christine Burns, MBE, MSc, BSc, CEng, MBCS, CITP,
Vice President, Press for Change

"Therapists working with transgender clients—and transgender readers, too—should find intriguing insights in this collection, a rich and varied array of informative and provocative stories of relationships testifying to the love that transgender people experience and the complexities of transgender lives. Whether naïve or sophisticated, the contributors are honest and forthright, stripping away the facades that so often obscure understanding. Love makes us all human."

Jamison Green, MFA
Postgraduate Researcher, Manchester Metropolitan University,
Author of Becoming a Visible Man

Trans People in Love

Trans People in Love

Tracie O'Keefe
Katrina Fox
Editors

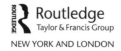
Routledge
Taylor & Francis Group

NEW YORK AND LONDON

First published 2008
by Routledge
270 Madison Ave, New York, NY 10016

Simultaneously published in the UK
by Routledge
2 Park Square, Milton Park, Abingdon, Oxon OX14 4RN

Routledge is an imprint of the Taylor & Francis Group, an informa business

Library of Congress Cataloging in Publication Data
  Trans People in Love / Tracie O'Keefe, Katrina Fox, editors.
    p. cm
  Includes bibliographical references and index.
  1. Transgenderism. 2. Transgender people-Biography. 3. Love. I.
O'Keefe, Tracie. II. Fox, Katrina.
  HQ77.7.T736 2007
  306.76'80922-dc22

                                                      2007045396

ISBN10: 0-7890-3571-5 (hbk)
ISBN10: 0-7890-3572-3 (pbk)
ISBN10: 0-20388-947-9 (ebk)

ISBN13: 978-0-7890-3571-4 (hbk)
ISBN13: 978-0-7890-3572-1 (pbk)
ISBN13: 978-0-20388-947-3 (ebk)

CONTENTS

ABOUT THE EDITORS

Tracie O'Keefe, DCH, is a clinical hypnotherapist, psychotherapist, counselor, and sex therapist, originally from London, England. Since 2001, she has lived and practiced in Sydney, Australia. She is a trans woman who transitioned over thirty-five years ago and now runs the Australian Health & Education Centre, Sydney. She is a member of the World Professional Association for Transgender Health (WPATH), Australian Association of Sex, Educators, Researchers and Therapists (ASSERT), and registered with the Psychotherapy and Counseling Federation of Australia (PACFA). Dr. O'Keefe is the author of many papers and articles on sex, gender, and sexuality diversity, co-author of *Trans-X-U-All: The Naked Difference*, the author of *Sex, Gender & Sexuality: 21st Century Transformations*, and the co-editor of *Finding the Real Me: True Tales of Sex & Gender Diversity*, an anthology of real-life stories by sex- and gender-diverse people. She is also the author of *Investigating Stage Hypnosis and Self-Hypnosis for Life: Mind, Body, and Spiritual Excellence*. In addition to being a clinician and writer, Dr. O'Keefe is also a passionate campaigner for the rights of sex- and gender-diverse people. She was a founding member of lobby group Sex and Gender Education (SAGE) in Australia (www.sageaustralia.org) where she serves on its steering committee and can often be found educating bureaucrats and government officials regarding discriminatory laws and policies against trans people. More info at www.tracieokeefe.com.

Katrina Fox is a freelance journalist, writing predominantly for the GLBTIQ press. She is the editor of *CHERRIE*, a monthly magazine for lesbian and queer women in Australia and writes regularly for *SX*, a weekly arts, news, and entertainment magazine for the GLBTIQ community in Sydney, including a column "Keeping Abreast". Her work has also appeared in *DIVA*, the UK's national lesbian magazine, and *Curve*, a U.S. national lesbian magazine. She is the co-author of *Trans-X-U-All: The Naked Difference*, the editor of *Sex, Gender & Sexuality*, and co-editor of *Finding the Real Me*. More info at www.katrinafox.com.

Trans People In Love

Contributors

Jacob Anderson-Minshall pens the weekly syndicated column *TransNation* which appears in LGBT papers from San Francisco to Boston. He and his wife Diane (editor of U.S. national lesbian magazine *Curve*) have been together for seventeen years. In 1994, the two co-founded *Girlfriends* magazine; they currently co-author the Blind Eye mystery series which premiered April 2007 with *Blind Curves*. They are also writing a relationship memoir about surviving transition which is due out in 2008. Find out more at anderson-minshall .com or e-mail Jacob at jake@trans-nation.org.

Martine Delaney lives with her partner, Jen, two dogs and six cats in a suburb of Hobart, capital of the island of Tasmania, the southernmost state of Australia. While Jen works to keep them all fed, Martine is presently busy seeking ways to become rich and famous, so they can afford to build a home on their bush block. Known in recent years as a "sex-change soccer star," Martine actually spends much of her time working as an unpaid advocate for trans rights and taking on anti-discrimination cases against secretive religious sects and conservative political parties. And she is truly enjoying loving Jen.

Orsekov Dan was born in 1982 in the small town of Kyrgyzstan in Russia. He spent half his life in the village where his mom lives. He wants to grow as a writer, artist, and photographer and is about to start art school. He is currently studying German, psychology, and journalism, and works with computers, which he describes as "quiet work where I have a lot of time for self-education." In the future he intends to write scientific work on moral tyranny and about the psychology of children aged eleven and twelve. His wife dreams of starting a school for gifted children, which is the couple's preparation for their future children.

Lee "Bridgett" Harrington is an eclectic performer, artist, model, spiritual, and erotic educator and gender radical from the U.S. She is the author of *Shibari You Can Use: Japanese Rope Bondage and Erotic Macramé*. Part of the international kink and sex-positive communities since 1995, hir stories make people laugh while showing you that eroticism can be as serious, sexy, or silly as you make it. Lee/Bridgett's writings and photography have appeared in numerous anthologies and magazines, and hir image has been seen everywhere from PlayBoy TV to the pages of *Skin Two* magazine. To learn more about Lee, visit www.PassionAndSoul.com.

Debra Hastings was born in a small country town in Australia. When she was sixteen, her family moved to Sydney where she quickly adapted to big-city life and discovered who and what she was. In 1990 she moved to London. She now has a career, a home of her own, friends of all genders and sexualities, and although still living in the male role, is legally married to the love of her life, a beautiful English lad called David. Debra is a vegetarian, into Goth metal, sci-fi, and all things new age. For further details check out www .myspace.com/debra323.

Jody Helfand has an MA in English and an MFA in Creative Writing and has written two books of poetry. His work has appeared in over thirty journals and magazines. His obsessions include moving from Hawaii to Vancouver, playing with his family, playing with his dogs, eating crab cakes at Bali By The Sea, Danzig, AFI, Sigur Ros, and carrot juice made from organic carrots. He is currently reading *Vampire Loves* by Joann Sfar. He is also hard at work on his memoir and is looking for a publisher. If you would like to contact him, send an e-mail to jhrose22@hotmail.com.

Monica F. Helms is originally from Arizona. She started her transition in June of 1997, and moved to Atlanta in 2000. She served on the board of several national and local GLBT organizations and is the President of the Transgender American Veterans Association (TAVA). Monica is also a published author, having written seven novels of which one has been published. She has written a regular column for *Transgender Tapestry* for six years, over twenty short stories, countless articles, and op-ed pieces for magazines and newspapers. One of her short stories, *The Phone of Plenty,* won third place in the 1993 Arizona Author's Contest.

Jordy Jones is a scholar, curator, multimedia artist, and community advocate. His work includes investigations of issues surrounding human bodies and their relationships to culture, technology, representation, and subject formation. He is a UC Chancellor's Fellow and a PhD candidate in Visual Studies and Critical Theory at the University of California, Irvine. His dissertation, *The Ambiguous I: Photography, Gender, Self,* addresses self-representation of gender and somatic ambiguity in photography. In the winter of 2008, he will be on the academic job market and will launch jordyjones.com.

Zayne Jones is thirty-four years old. His partner's name is Tami Wheeler and he has a twelve-year-old daughter, whose name is Kylie. Zayne currently lives in Sacramento, California. He started his transition in August of 2005, and identifies as transgender, along with many other aspects of his personality. He chooses to be open and honest about himself because he would like to think that he could make a difference. He currently attends school with the goal of becoming a registered nurse. In the summer of 2008 he and Tami and are getting married.

Kayla Karstens is a professional jazz guitarist from South Africa and has supported herself as a musician and traveled the world for eighteen years. She is planning on releasing a CD of original jazz. Inspired by her trans experience, she is writing a script and composing the musical score for a stage musical. She underwent her gender reassignment surgery and facial feminization surgery at the Suporn Clinic in Thailand in April 2007. Kayla is deeply overwhelmed with joy and elation at finally transitioning and is interested in getting involved with trans-related activism. She can be contacted by e-mail at kayla_jesica_karstens@yahoo.co.uk.

Nick Laird lives in Glasgow, Scotland with his partner Mark and their dog Floyd. Nick is out and proud to be trans and believes gender inequality is best viewed through a trans lens. He works doing training and community development for a Scottish executive-funded project to support LGBT inclusion in the National Health Service in Scotland, based at the Glasgow LGBT Centre. Nick loves spending time with Mark and with his sister, brother, niece, nephews, dad and the rest of his family. He also loves creative writing, long daydreaming walks with the dog, the occasional cocktail, and a good book.

Isaac Lindstrom is a twenty-six-year-old trans guy who is a foreign adoptee and lives in Sweden. Studying at the university is important to him. His special interests are questions concerning views of life. Theories about body, sex, gender, and race are his main focus. Currently he is working on an application for graduate studies while he is studying philosophy, and he will be a very dedicated scientist. He is also into trans activism in one of the world's oldest gay liberation movements (RFSL) despite the fact that he is not gay.

Stenton Mackenzie is a graduate student of forensic anthropology at the University of Dundee in Scotland. As the fruit of English and Scottish bohemian loins, this Canadian-raised hybrid is a queer trans man with a taste for the irreverent, the rebellious and the righteous. Some of his favorite things are Guinness, boxer motorcycles, really nice marijuana, dogs, leather, gardens, books, water, and frolicsome sex.

Nickolas J. McDaniel is an FTM who is an active participant in the trans movement. An eloquent speaker and compelling writer, Nick has appeared in documentaries and publications regarding transsexualism. Over the past five years he has spoken to numerous audiences in an educational capacity on such topics as transsexualism and male sexual abuse. Currently he is a member of the American Association of Sex Educators, Counselors, and Therapists (AASECT) and is pursuing certification as a sex therapist and gender specialist. He is proud of being both a man and a transsexual.

Dr. Rusty Mae Moore lives in Brooklyn and upstate New York with her three nest mates. She has been a professor of international business for the past thirty-five years, and has been a tenured faculty member of Hofstra University on Long Island since 1982. Rusty has three grown children and one grandchild who also live in Brooklyn. She and Chelsea Goodwin have been the co-mothers of Transy House, a collective home for queer people in transition for the past twelve years. Rusty's hobbies include cycling, travel, woodworking, photography, folk singing, and writing. Her blog is at http://green frogcafe.blogspot.com.

Joseph J. Nutini is a self-identified trans man, activist, queer, poly-amorous, spiritualist, and future famous writer. He has a bachelor's degree from the Univeristy of Arizona in Women's Studies and a Master's in Social Work from Arizona State. He enjoys spending time hiking in beautiful Tucson, Arizona when he is not practicing social work. Currently Joe is working on two books: One that is his story as a twenty-something trans man (he is now twenty-six); and another that is about polyamorous relationships and theory.

Andrés Ignacio Rivera Duarte is a Chilean transsexual man who was born on January 27, 1964 and lives in Rancagua, Chile. He is the founder and president of the first organization of transsexual men in Chile, and is a professor and university lecturer, advisor, and consultant. Andrés has accomplished the unprecedented in his country: the creation of a system of free or publicly-subsidized care for transsexual persons at the Rancagua Hospital, so that they can be diagnosed and can receive hormonal and surgical treatment. He has also carried out projects for sex workers, educating them on their human rights, on the transmission of sexual diseases including HIV/AIDS, and on the prevention of drug and alcohol abuse.

Vidal Rousso was born in Latvia. In the summer of 2005, he moved to Sweden, to be with his girlfriend, Christine. Several of Vidal's early stories were published in the Latvian gay newspaper, *10%*. Most of his creativity finds its expression through shows though; he has worked as a choreographer in Riga, and has performed in Riga, Stockholm, and London. He is interested in photography, rock music, art films, Native American philosophy, and experience. You can read more about him at www.vidalrousso.com.

Carmen Rupe. In her own words, Carmen, who is of Maori origin, says: "Just as my name Carmen suggests, I am a trans woman of great passion. But more than that, I am also a bird of paradise who color-fully tries to light up each place I go. You can't miss me with my high red hair, glamorous clothes, and sparkling adornments, but I am more than the window dressing. Now in my seventieth year, I have, since the 1950s, been at the forefront of gay and trans liberation both in my native New Zealand and Australia. I never hid who or what I was but celebrated and shared my many differences, and oh, how they loved me . . . even when they scorned me."

Joelle Ruby Ryan is currently completing her PhD in American Culture Studies at Bowling Green State University, Ohio. Her research areas include trans identity, feminism, film/media, fat studies, and sex work. She has taught university courses in women's studies, ethnic studies, American studies, English composition and LGBT Studies. She is the producer of the autobiographical video *TransAmazon* (2003) and the author of *Gender Quake: Poems* (2005). She has been active in LGBT, feminist, anti-racist, and anti-war causes since the early 1990s and is a frequent speaker at conferences and community groups. You can find out more about Joelle at www.joellerubyryan .com.

Armanda Scheidegger was born in Switzerland as a boy but lived with the thought: "Why can't I live like other girls and wear a pretty skirt?" As she grew older, she carried the hope of being a wife and a mother happily in her heart. "Every day the unrealizable desire to apply my femininity and my social skills was torturing me, but working as a nurse allowed me to take care of my patients and give them some kind of comfort," she says. "When I was forty years old I had the courage to talk to my family and to my friends about my transsexuality and the difficulties that come along with it."

Susan Stryker is an independent scholar and filmmaker who lives and works in San Francisco. Her work includes *Gay by the Bay: A History of Queer Culture in San Francisco, Queer Pulp, The Transgender Studies Reader,* and the film *Screaming Queens: The Riot at Compton's Cafeteria.*

Gypsey Teague is branch head of Clemson University's Gunnin Architecture Library. She is also a nationally recognized teacher, writer, and lecturer on the subject of transgenderism and she is the only male-to-female transgender faculty member at any South Carolina state university. As a member of the women's studies department at Clemson, she teaches transgender and gender subjects to both graduate and undergraduate students. Gypsey is the author of three novels, the first of which, *The Life and Deaths of Carter Falls,* was an American Library Association Stone Award nominee for GLBT fiction. She is also the editor of the recently published textbook on male-to-female transgenders, *The New Goddess: Transgender Women in the Twenty-First Century.*

TinyBelly is a pre-op transsexual and a graduate student in Taiwan. In her leisure time she devotes herself to LGBTQ and sex workers' rights movements. "Gay and lesbian liberation in my country has been quite active in recent years, but the transgender movement is just on the starting line," she says. "We have a gay pride parade every year around October. If you come to join the parade, you may see me there." To contact TinyBelly, e-mail tinybelly@gmail.com.

Erica Zander is a fifty-four-year-old male-to-female transsexual from Sweden who lives with her partner of thirty-five years. Easily blending in with her hippie style "transvestism," her cross-dressing was soon a natural part of their everyday life. Aged thirty, and a father of two, she took an unexpected trans time-out, only to realize, fifteen years later, that she was really a gay woman. "Of course you are," her wife said. Always having been quite public with her situation, Erica is still not all that comfortable with the fact the people still recognize the couple from an interview they did on national television in 2002. Her autobiography *TransActions* was published in 2003. Visit Erica's Web site at www.ericazander.com.

Foreword

Trans People in Love is a sometimes erotic, always respectful homage to love, both magical and tragical. Maybe this book was given to you by a transgender person who wants you to know that they are loved and loving. Maybe this book was a gift from someone who loves a transgender person and they want you to know how thrilled that makes them. You know how good it feels when a friend or family member is in love and you feel happy for them? That's how this book made us feel: happy for our family. Not too many people really get us, beyond ourselves. And once you really get us, it turns out you're one of us. So if you bought this book yourself, just because you were curious, welcome to our world.

There are a great many voices in this book. Voices from the days when there was no word, "transgender," and the general public only ever heard about the white, middle-class, and middle-aged "men who wanted to be women." Those trannies were mostly refined and proper and their role models were "real ladies." But we can be a whole lot of genders, and no matter what gender we decide we are, there always seems to be someone out there to love us. No matter what gender we'd like our lover to be, no matter how gender gets defined, we can find a lover who's the gender of our dreams. We can be or find a gentle lady, and we can be or find a transgender stone butch man. And the varieties of sex are as numerous as the genders. There's religious sex, and sacrilegious sex—and the religious images extend from God the Father to the holy whore of Babylon. There's monogamy, polyamory, and orgasmic celibacy.

But this book is not just about gender and sex, it's also about love—love in all its glory and all its pain. There's young love, there's long love tried and true, and there's love that burns out in a blaze of glory. There's love when one lover is older—maybe by a lot—and love when they're the same age. There's love when one lover is younger than the other—sometimes a lot younger. There are couples who

Trans People In Love

start out heterosexual and end up as a pair of lesbians! There are couples who are heterosexual men and women and end up as two gay men! There are couples in this book who start out lesbian, and end up as "man" and "woman" but they're not even close to heterosexual and they like it that way. Honest, all of that is in this book someplace!

Our trannie love and love for trannies crosses lines of class and sexuality. We love each other in suits and ties and skirts and pantyhose, but also in denim and leather, and with whips and scalpels. There are genders in this book that most of the world has never heard about … yet. And there are people in the world who love each and every one of them. And that's the point of the book: we have our love stories, too. And sometimes they're magic, and sometimes they're tragic, but it's a sweet kind of love that not too many people know about. You're about to be one of the very first who get to find out.

If you're feeling particularly daring and you'd like to know for yourself what love in another gender might feel like, try putting yourself in the shoes of the narrator of each chapter in this book. Then ask, "What gender am I? Why am I that gender? And if I am that gender, will anyone love me?" The answer to that last question is a big, resounding YES! Yes, there's love for you, no matter what your gender is. That's the message of this sweet collection of vulnerability, pride, and sex positivism: there's delight in every word and potential for delight in every gender.

Trans People in Love is a book that will go a long way toward healing our wounds as sex and gender outlaws. Thank you to Tracie O'Keefe and Katrina Fox for putting this together, and to all the brave, wonderfully gendered people who've written in here. We're proud to be family with you.

Love and kisses,
Kate Bornstein & Barbara Carrellas

Preface

Millions of people throughout the world are trans—that is, they are transsexual, transexed, transgender, transvestites (cross-dressers), some of whom are also intersexed. This is a first ever volume of stories by trans people, from all different parts of the world, who are in love and tell us in their own voices about how they forge and maintain loving relationships with a significant other or others. The trans people in this book are in or have been in a diverse range of relationships—straight, gay, bisexual, queer, polyamorous. Some are male-to-female (MTF) and female-to-male (FTM) and others sit outside the male-female gender binary.

This exciting project took seven years to come to fruition. It began with a pilot study of trans people and their partners who were kind enough to open their hearts and let us peer within. The pilot study revealed the importance of partners' attitudes in those relationships. When we put out our call for trans people to submit their real-life experiences of love and relationships, we were delighted to receive a wonderful collection of powerful and moving stories, which present the trials, tribulations, and triumphs experienced by trans people in their various relationships. Some of the stories are challenging, sexy, and passionate, others are funny, joyful, and sad.

We, the editors, are one transexed woman who is a therapist and sexologist working with trans people, and her female lover who is a journalist and editor. At the time of this book's publication we will have been in a committed relationship for fifteen years. We ourselves have had an incredibly rewarding time that has added to both our lives in so many positive ways. Much of the world we know, however, still sees all trans people as sad, lonely, hopeless, and unlovable rejects. This volume resoundingly puts that myth to bed forever and shows that trans people can love and be in love passionately.

There is no comment on the stories or analyzing of them. We simply present them in their raw, unadulterated form. This allows the richness of the contributors' experiences to teach us about their incredible ingenuity as they negotiate a love experience with bodies and self-images that are transient and fluid. Never before have so many trans voices publicly spoken of loving in such frank and honest ways.

What is also so very clear about these stories is that they are all very different and that in itself demonstrates how resourceful we can all be as human beings. In reading them, one is left with a deep sense of respect for each contributor, knowing that often love comes in the face of profound public prejudice. They have shown amazing willingness to tell us about their most vulnerable of all experiences—of opening up their hearts and letting another person inside in an act of falling in love.

Read and enjoy!

Tracie O'Keefe & Katrina Fox
June 2007

Acknowledgments

We would like to say a huge thank-you to all the contributors who bravely allowed us to peer into their lives and hearts, reviewing first-hand the mechanics, highs, lows, and adventures of their experiences of being in love.

Many thanks are also due to the friends of some of the non-English-speaking contributors who voluntarily translated stories into English, as well as all the gay, lesbian, bisexual, trans, intersex and queer (GLBTIQ) groups and individuals, especially Cassie Biggs and Frank Zhao, who helped spread the call out for contributions, thereby ensuring this book reflects international voices and perspectives.

We are very grateful to our publishers, the Haworth Press who were farsighted enough to take on this project, proving once again that publishing can be as much about social consciousness as it is about profit. Particular thanks go to our book program editor, Eli Coleman, and to Robert Owen who patiently answered all our queries.

We would like to thank our foreword writers, renowned gender theorist Kate Bornstein (*Gender Outlaw, My Gender Workbook, Hello Cruel World*) whose contributions to the gender debate are always inspiring, down-to-earth and humorous, and her partner, Barbara Carrellas whose book *Urban Tantra* is the most GLBTIQ-friendly on the subject and offers some fantastic suggestions to spice up the love lives of all.

Living and loving contributes to the people we are and have become, so we'd like to thank all our past loves and lovers for the ride.

Last, but by no means least, we'd like to thank our tabby cat Gabrielle (and her sister, Xena, who passed away two years ago), for reminding us that love and family come in a multitude of forms.

1

Switcheroo

Stenton Mackenzie

I married her twice. She divorced me twice. The first time brutally, the second time, very coldly. The love we shared was anything but cold. I was pinned quite forcefully by it into a union, that became for me, the very fabric of my life. I learned more than I ever thought it might be possible to learn from another; I still mourn her absence, I still dream of her, vividly, strangely, hauntingly. I sometimes wish that she had died, imagining this would change the nature of my memory, and my gaping sense of loss. Perhaps her death would render romantic what really had not been a romantic affair—intense, transforming, dissembling, chaotic, exciting, dangerous, all of these—but not romantic.

My existence consisted of my life before her, my life with her, and now this. I am still "recovering" as the white coats put it, doing remarkably well they say, but who are they to comment on my progress out of the abyss? Paid to be impartial, trained to measure and weigh, sift, and objectify. This of course is why we go to them, for their "impartiality," that exact quality lacking in the emergent, raw, writhing pain of separation.

We knew each other so well it often astonished us. The intimacy was like a drug and it makes her absence so painful still. It is as if a piece of me is missing. She and I had a symbiosis, an ability to understand what the other was thinking and feeling. We could finish each other's sentences; we were barometers of each other's fears and desires. We had chemistry; moments of brilliant repartee, people would sip—no, guzzle—off our interaction, attracted by the doubling of charisma and the giddy, infectious intoxication of being utterly in love. We flaunted our spark, daring others to harness their own electricity. Our love was larger, grander, more enthralling than either of us had experienced with another. Our intensity fed upon itself, fueling a higher and higher sensitivity to each other, which was irresistible, like a narcosis, which upon removal felt like a little death.

We came close to dying together in the early days: an Alpha Romeo convertible she had taken great delight in my encouraging her to buy slipped away from the black ice on the tarmac of a railway overpass on an early December day not long after we were first married. It catapulted down a sixty-foot embankment, twisting and pivoting diagonally, and landed upside down, rocking on a roll bar I had insisted on having installed only weeks before. The convertible rested on an enormous tree stump measuring some six to eight feet across, and we swung suspended in seat belts beneath the roll bar, which prevented us from being flattened like bugs. As the car left the bridge and took flight, she reached over, took my hand, and said very simply, "I love you." The memory is crystal clear. In those molasses-like moments before the car finally struck the earth at the bottom, with a sound like an-end-of-the-world-explosion, we thought we were going to die.

Oddly enough, the edgy drama of those moments did not bond us together; our individual recovery differed—I adjusted more poorly to the confusion and fear, which is part and parcel of healing after head injuries, while she was impatient to get back to work and put it behind her. I wallowed. She was cross and tired.

The ambulance attendants, admissions staff, and nurses who subjected us to untender mercies for the three days we spent in the hospital were disenchanted by our attempts to remain together in the emergency ward. They wanted to separate us onto different floors; mostly I think to avoid the discomfort of nursing two lesbians who were obvious in their love for each other. Homophobic nurses armed with large needles were cruel in their dispensing of power. My wife rose from her bed, staggering drunkenly from head trauma, dragging a saline drip and pole in her wake, and in loud, uncompromising tones declared we would only be separated over some nurse's dead body—"Whose was is going to be?" I lost consciousness again somewhere in the negotiation between a small squadron of grim-faced emergency staff and my protector. Ultimately, we were rescued by the impressive domination of my mother's latest husband, an ex-Major General who was not going to be disobeyed by a few insubordinate nurses. The General had the final say, returning subsequently to transport us from the inhospitable malignancy of the emergency ward.

* * *

The Freudian and post-Freudian position that all our experiences of love relations are ultimately and finally a result of the initial bond with our mothers is not far off the mark. My mother was a romantic—in all relationships, not just with men—and it was her downfall. The word "downfall" is now oddly antiquarian, invoking a Western idea of courtly love born out of the dark ages of Europe and ending in a fizzle sometime before the first World War. It resonates strongly with the mysteries of fate, a beguiling concept in itself, particularly for romantics, who rely heavily on its intricacies in deciphering the whys and wherefores of their loves, losses, and near misses.

I felt romanced in the beginning. She pursued me with a certainty that was a bit shocking. I was young—only twenty-two to her thirty-three. She seemed altogether sure of herself, perhaps a bit bossy. I did not mind that. It was reassuring. Her certainty swept all those before it. She charmed my mother, to whose home I had recently returned in a hasty and undignified retreat from my first marriage, which had ended in a graceless and unchivalrous infidelity on my part. I had schlepped home with a lover, possessing in her youth equally graceless tendencies and a leaning toward the bottle and bitterness. I left this uncouth companion to her own devices one night and went to a lezzie dance at a local hall. I was trying to pull up my socks, to pull myself out of an aimless lethargy that had overcome me. I went out to "put on the dog" I suppose. The unwarranted ungratefulness of the companion rescued from the dank and wasted fundamentalist population of a Canadian province that shall remain unnamed was taking a toll. She and I shared a room in a condemned Catholic Chapel as we huddled against the most savage winter experienced in that locale in one hundred and twenty-five years. Of course that *would* have been the year that my first wife and I chose to make our great escape from the incestuous lesbian community in which we had met. We drove many thousands of miles in an adventurous, but as it turned out, uninspired choice, to face a winter of catastrophic proportions.

Perversely, my return to the community I had suddenly and disastrously left, led me straight into the arms of my second wife, to whom my first wife had introduced me to three years earlier. No one except us seemed particularly happy with this new turn of events—not the rescued girlfriend, not my first wife, nor the current wife of my then to-be second wife. It was messy, but my new lover cared not a bit. She bedded me and promptly moved me into the "family" home which consisted, prior to my arrival, of herself, her wife, her son, two large dogs, and a couple of cats. Everyone disapproved. I was witless, carried along on a tide of lust and the vague sense of having escaped, yet again, an unfortunate assemblage of boring, unattractive, and seemingly futureless details of my life.

I have always claimed I fell in love with her the afternoon of our first introduction, myself a tender nineteen years of age. She halfheartedly scoffed at this assertion in the way women do when they are secretly pleased that you could have, or might have, felt such a powerful and instant attraction, even if they suspect you are wishfully and retroactively doctoring the story. I do know I felt something I had never felt before that afternoon, as she poured tea from her big Brown Betty. It lingered. It drew me in. I was curious. And I was conscious of her curiosity. I often return in my mind to our first meeting, rooting and digging for the edges of that feeling, and finding, in spite of it having no clear borders or no distinct definition, that it remained compelling.

As the trans man I am now, I look back, trying to identify moments which possess a significance that only exist in the retrospect of a special and unique vantage point. She always liked my maleness. She had no hesitation in saying that. She was almost proud of my maleness, adamant in stating that it was a strong element in the sex between us. I was androgynous. Half of the time, unless I opened my mouth, people mistook me for a male. My hips are small, my shoulders wide. My face was angular, and big-nosed, my expressions and gestures masculine. My hair was dead straight and often cut very short. I walked with a swagger, spoke in direct phrases, and had a direct gaze. I never said much.

She said the reason I so often won the disapproval of lesbians was because I was so male. I had emerged in the 1970s andro-clone season when all lesbians wore plaid shirts, no one admitted to using dildos, let alone a strap-on, and the politics of sex equated penetration with rape and patriarchy. So we did not penetrate. Bollocks. We did, we just didn't admit it. Those politics also said femmes did not exist. To be a butch was slightly more acceptable, but still begging for exclusion. I was excommunicated many times over.

She and I started to wear leather; we flirted with the style but not much of the content of the S/M world for which the likes of Pat(rick) Califia were (and still are) resoundingly condemned. We shared a mutual fascination with Carole Pope's raw sexuality and uncontained identity; we spent money on drugs—cocaine, grass, hash—on good scotch, on nights in hotel rooms with room service and nice linen. We celebrated sex. We dug in and got our faces dirty. We rolled like unconstrained pigs in the turbulence of our fights, which were many and damaging, and in the aftermath of those emotional holocausts we slathered on the salve of combustible sexual diversions. It was heady stuff. I still have the scar on my shoulder where she bit clean through the epidermis into my deltoid muscle during the throes of an orgasm. I know she will not forget when I took her for the first time with my fist, quite spontaneously, up against the wall on the floor in the suite at Long Beach, and she sucked my fist in so deeply that I was lodged halfway to my elbow as she spasmed around my forearm, completely helpless in the necessity of surrender.

When my clit took off under the effects of the testosterone she was impressed and excited. She was horrified at the savagery of the bilateral mastectomy, which never looks terribly presentable in the early stages of recovery. She was there briefly after the first of my chest reconstructions—we had separated for the second time at that point— she said she mourned the loss of my breasts and declared the surgery a mutilation. She felt differently about my micro-phallus. In some of my darkest moments when I have longed for the intimacy and the intensity our sexual dialogue forged (ironically, most particularly during the last few disintegrating years of our marriage), I would torture myself with the memory of her, mouth full with my little phallus, slurping and groaning as she sucked me, saying in a breathless voice, "God, it's so big." I felt like a king, and she like my queen, and not just the king and queen of a porn movie, which in all fairness is laughingly what that scene brings to mind. All I heard was the desire in her voice—desire for me, for what I had become, for what I was becoming. And I rejoiced. The biggest fear that transsexuals face is that no one will ever love them or desire them again as a result of the changes wrought by surgery and hormones. That afternoon I knew I had touched a deep level of want in her, and that want was for me, at that moment, in that form, in all my "hugeness." And I was happy.

That, however, was not to last. It was a brief respite amidst the tail end of the second divorce, and is all the more poignant because of a juxtaposition with the agony of the second, final separation. I will now make the bold claim that it was not my transition that ended the marriage. It was, as that common catchphrase of straight divorce documents in years past went—irreconcilable differences. Differences potent enough to eventually destroy the fragile bond that initially drew us together. She may deny it, but I truly believe that my being a trannie was really just a blip in the chart relative to our other dilemmas. The problems and the errors of judgement we made along the way seem to have little to do with something, in my case, as explicable as gender displacement. I think in her heart of hearts, she actually had a great deal of sympathy and understanding of my predicament. But it was perhaps in some ways the perfect excuse for drawing an end to what had become a very painful and dangerous relationship. The difficulty for me has always been that there was so much that was joyful in our union. It was almost as if our love led another life, a separate existence entirely from the squalor and immaturity of our fights, the struggles for control, and the relentless acquisition of layers of damage of which we were intimately aware, but unable to prevent.

* * *

There were no ceremonies for our first or second union, unlike the present gay trend toward public and legal formalities. We celebrated in our own, private way, walking a favorite beautiful beach at night, wandering into the water's edge, hand in hand, kissing, murmuring, promising. She paid for a honeymoon holiday in San Francisco, a hotel in the gay ghetto, dinners of sushi and champagne. I laid on the nude beach far too long one afternoon and roasted so excessively that I had to retreat to the double bed in the hotel with ice cubes and the blinds drawn for a couple of days, and she complained I wasn't much fun in such a condition. Sex was out of the question. To make matters worse, my eyelids swelled shut, rendering me blind for a short time.

In those days I had a twenty-eight inch waist; she delighted in buying the tightest jeans I could squeeze into, and encouraged me into baths of hot water, insisting I wear the jeans on my body until they dried, thus ensuring the eventual fit would have the maximum amount of sex appeal. She loved being the older of our pairing. At this point she was thirty-four to my twenty-three, and this titillated her. She luxuriated in the mystique of the older woman seducing the younger. She played happily to my youth and naivety. And I was naive.

We explored San Francisco (SF) on our honeymoon, returning another time on two motorcycles with her eight-year-old son—my stepson—who rode mostly behind me since she judged me the better rider and therefore the safer bet for his survival. We relished SF even though it was long past its prime by then. By the late 1980s the Pride parade was a pathos-filled mix of the healthy, flamboyantly pinkest-of-the-pink, and gaunt faggots gamely lugging their oxygen tanks behind weakened, scarred bodies. In 1983 my lover and I revelled in the queer counter-culture of the city, exploring Castro and the Tenderloin at night with an equal share of touristic voyeurism and genuine feelings of belonging. We wore our black head-to-foot leather, jiving on the camaraderie of the other leather freaks on the pavement and in numerous holes-in-walls.

We found a bar that made such an impression on me, that sometimes the memory feels imagined rather than real. The Oasis was a large venue, inhabited by what, to my rural, small-town self, was surely the crème de la crème of the hip sexual and social outlaws of SF. It was sophisticated, utterly relaxing, and totally absorbing. The music was sublime, rooms segued one into another, people wandered, talked, danced, and slithered from group to group; we felt as though we had come home. I remember clutching one another in our excitement as if it had been created just for us. Years later we sought it out again, but it had, of course, changed radically and we were out of place and pointedly unwelcome.

But that night we were in heaven. Out back a swimming pool was surrounded by lights and people sauntering, vibing, and, to our intense delight, smoking marijuana. It was the first time we had tripped across a public bar or club in which this was permitted and indeed, seemed de rigueur. We lit up and roamed amongst the crowd, congratulating ourselves on our good fortune, mentally etching the mood and environment into our beings, knowing such an encounter would not soon come along again, if ever. The Oasis fed our sense of solidarity—as if all our wildest hopes of how people might socialize if only they had the necessary imagination. For my lover it was a whiff of her memories of the 1960s, for me it was what I had always been missing, but could never really envision.

In San Francisco we met our first flesh-and-blood trannie, a male to female (MTF) of extraordinary insight, intelligence, and gentle sensibility. She (DB) drank scotch with us in the hotel bar and shared tales of transitional adventure. She was fascinating. I was intrigued, and so was my lover. Why it did not occur to me then that such a thing, in reverse, was possible for me, I will never understand. It would take another ten years before it swam into my perception as an answer to my discomfort at my position in the world. I don't say *the* answer, because nothing is ever that simple.

Our new friend was midway through surgical transition, fabulously dressed, and projecting an assured and dignified presence. She was sad about the losses in her life which gender reassignment visits upon the transgressors of "normality;" wives, husbands, children, jobs and careers are all grist to the mill for many transsexuals, and sometimes, I think recovery from the loss of significant others is an insurmountable barrier to contentment in a new life. She continued with her business (refrigeration) and mused at the confusion some of her customers suffered when she showed up to deal with business in person rather than over the phone. Her voice never rose to a convincing female pitch, and I think she continued much of her business over the phone in her old male persona for the sake of convenience. At any rate, DB was positively inspiring and she will forever have a place in my heart. If there is any justice in this world, one day I will run into her at a trannie conference, and we will sit down to an irreverent chinwag over a bottle of good scotch to weep tears of trannie camaraderie over the various tragedies of love and transition.

My wife and I occasionally talked about our encounter with DB over the years, and in relation to that, I think she was both bemused and shocked with the complete lack of hesitation that described my transition. It did not actually *require* a decision on my part; as soon as I understood that it was possible, I made an appointment with a physician, knowing somehow there would be little resistance to my request and that I would encounter little denial from the gender "experts." And, it was relatively simple in retrospect. I told them who I was; I related a life history resulting in a diagnosis as a "True Transsexual, class 4" without having to tell any lies, and after being very firm in my refusal of psychotherapeutic counselling, started my "real life test." I took testosterone, had various surgeries, and here I am . . . for the most part, a happy, well-balanced, life-embracing trans man. I often fend off compliments offered about my "bravery," saying that on the contrary, no bravery was ever called for as I suffered not even a microsecond of doubt. The knowledge that changing my gender appearance to line up with what most people perceived me as already, and what I felt more aligned and comfortable with in my head, was my release.

I don't think my wife ever really accepted or comprehended how little thought was necessary for me to embrace the change, and as a result, was perhaps understandably suspicious of the speed of the process. I think she felt left out, as if she were not an important part of my rationale in making such a catastrophic reengagement with my (and our) world.

I have to admit I did not know my sexual orientation could undergo a change in direction, but nothing in life is perfect, and although it does pose certain challenges I had not foreseen, I am not derailed by this mysterious and compelling divergence of my sexuality. It is certainly interesting and I often feel it constitutes a sort of quirky bonus prize in the entire continuum of who I am becoming. Now I can hear you thinking ... how could this guy ever expect anything but the dissolution of his marriage to a woman who identified as a lesbian, when, on top of being a transitioning transsexual, his orientation swings from gynophilic to androphilic?

She and I were on the rocks long before transition was a gleam in my eye. At first, our ideas appeared to be much the same, but as I matured and became more independent and as she struggled with demons of her own, it became more and more apparent that we did not share compatible world perspectives, even when agreeing to disagree. One of us had to sacrifice herself on the altar of the relationship or we had to separate. There was no other way, except our mutual destruction. The change that quite coincidentally arrived on my doorstep could do nothing to affect these larger issues.

The raging irony which afflicts me still is my suspicion that she would have made a great FTM! And that we would have made a wonderful queer trans man couple. In all fairness, there are more than a few dykes I have met over the years who certainly qualify as likely candidates. Indeed when I look back, I can think of many who could have been nothing else. So many of us did not know it was possible. And still don't. Perhaps I am utterly wrong about my former wife— but the romantic in me thirsts for the siren song of fantasy. I wonder what it might have been like to have my lover join me at that same edge, the edge of our, rather than just my, precipice; to launch ourselves, hand in hand, gendernauts and lovers . . . together.

I make no apologies for admitting to such daydreams, despite the fact that she is not actually here to disagree or comment—to do so would imply there is something wrong or shameful in being transgendered. Other couples have done it; tandem transitions will happen here and there, now and again. We were not destined for such synchrony. We were righteous in our love, in our claims upon each other. We drank from a reservoir of the most intense, glorious, and torturous experience that humans can share. She is still a part of me, a part I no longer wish to have erased from my perception so that I may find peace. I am both surrounded and enclosed with memory, but free to love again, and also to continue to love her in myself. To feel inseparable from another being is not to be a cripple; it is not as simple as being bound. Metaphors inadequate to the task crowd upon my brain and heart, which has grown several sizes larger from loving her.

2

My Desire to Be All Woman

Armanda Scheidegger

I was born in the "home for single mothers" in Hergiswil, Switzerland on September 3, 1950. The name my mother gave me was Armin, which means "savior of the poor." Before that, my mother had a short affair with a man called Bruno who already had a daughter and a son of his own with another woman. He withheld this information until my mother was pregnant. She felt deceived and separation was inevitable.

The first four years of my life I spent in the care of my aunt Marie and my uncle Ruedi in Rorschach, along with their sons Peter and Rolf. I was wholly accepted and my relationship with the boys was deeply harmonic. In order to make ends meet, my mother worked in Zurich as a maid and a waitress.

When I was four, my mother married her boyfriend Willi Scheidegger, who became a very kind and interesting adoptive father to me. Thus, we moved to Dietikon, where I spent an ideal youth. Before I entered grammar school I was enlisted in a mixed kindergarten, where I could do handicrafts, play with dolls, and create landscapes in the sand pit. During the afternoons our neighbor Mrs. Fuchs looked after me, since my mother was still working back then.

When I was six, I had a formative experience, which enhanced my desire to realize girlish pleasures. One day after kindergarten, at around four o'clock, I saw a red dress hanging at Mrs. Fuchs' sideboard. It had a white collar. Mrs. Fuchs noticed my interest and asked me whether I'd like to try it on. I nodded and Mrs. Fuchs handed it over to me, and without hesitation I got out of my sweater and my pants and put on the cute little skirt. Without saying a word, Mrs. Fuchs took me by the hand, led me to her mirror and I was able to admire myself from head to toe. I felt totally happy in this dress, and I almost melted at the thought of becoming a girl one day. Mrs. Fuchs started grinning and said: "You wear this skirt very nicely. I believe you want to be a girl." Her words confirmed my deepest desires. Before I left for home, I had to take off the skirt and I couldn't hold back my tears.

At the age of thirteen, I passed a dance test and was allowed to join a ballet school with girls and boys of the same age. For about a year we practiced a Hungarian folk dance intensely. From the girls I learned how to put on make-up and to do my hair, as well as the dancing expression. We performed at several events in our city and happily enjoyed our successes in front of an enthusiastic crowd. I had many precious encounters with the girls at that time and I was fascinated by their behavior. In the eighth grade, I had my first profound friendship with a girl. I found her wonderful in her charisma and very feminine in her shape. Her torso appeared slim, and her breasts slightly developed; her hips round and strong. She wore mainly skirts in warm colors, in a well-flowing contrast to her blouse or pullover. We went to the same class and I regarded her as my girl-idol. We shared the same ideas about a lot of things, talked about our goals, and about how to achieve happiness by having a family and raising kids. Due to our upbringing and our lack of courage our liaison was limited to a platonic relationship, filled with great sincerity and sunny laughing. Yet, already during school, our friendship dissolved.

In my first post-graduate education I learned how to be a tiler. This took me three years of working with linoleum, carpets, and plastic. This kind of tough work did not correspond with my own talents at all. With all my heart, I was looking for a job that would make use of my feminine caring for my fellow men. In the meantime, I still worked as a manual laborer, yet with a different employer, and I hoped to find a new challenge with my education as a nurse.

In the same year I had my first love affair with Barta (not her real name). She was a little bit younger than me and unfortunately abandoned her education as a nurse without a diploma. She didn't have an ideal upbringing and she possessed hardly any self-esteem or joy for life. Pretty soon she meant a lot to me and I cherished her openness to accept my advice and to put it to good use. In regards to love and sexuality, we desired each other and mainly enjoyed kissing and stroking. The usual kind of lust one feels for the coitus has been weakened up to this day; as an "anonymous woman" my life is full of compulsion; I wish to be desired as a woman, by men. All the time I must prove my manhood, and my biggest desire to "be a woman" must be suppressed. The anxiety coming out of this kind of double life leaves its traces. Is there someone out there who is that special person I can trust?

Shortly before Barta and I got married in 1973 she got her degree in home care. A wonderful time, two years later our first daughter was born. Sensing the child through Barta's warm skin overwhelmed me. Daughter Rebekka's birth offered a spontaneous connection to support the child in her development with all my love. All children are unique and are in need of warmth and security. The good working conditions in 1975 allowed me to get an education as a psychiatric nurse. From then on I had a lot of energy to bring out all my female talents, by taking care of the patients with psychosomatic diseases.

In the years from 1976 to 1978 two more healthy daughters were born, Sarah and Bettina. Barta was facing great challenges. She was very kindly doing all her housework, especially taking care of the three girls, and I helped her as well as I could. As parents we decided to enjoy the status quo and to refrain from having more children, due to financial and personal reasons. Barta refused to be sterilized, in case we were to separate one day and she wanted to have children with another man. Thus, I had to undergo a vasectomy and have my spermatic cord dissected. In my thoughts I also desired to have my penis amputated, which would bring me closer to being a woman.

Before Bettina's birth my wife told me that she wanted another man who could offer a more fulfilling sex life with her. There was nothing lacking in my role as a caring and loving husband, but she was looking for something else.

I was happy to finish my education with a degree in 1978 and that from then on I'd be able to share my strength with the needy. Working as a nurse gave me a totally new sense of value and motivation. I felt like a woman without changing my outfit, except for the feminine aprons, which we had to wear out of hygienic reasons. As a counselor I was often asked to share my life experiences with my co-workers and students, even on the most intimate subjects. Also, my knowledge, which I gained through literature, courses, and talks with patients, allowed me to give useful information on personal development, relationships, diseases, and euthanasia.

I got a different job in 1990 where I met a former co-worker of mine, Verna, who had just finished an education in nursing service. She spent her private life with her grown-up children who enjoyed their own relationships. When Verna and I both worked the early shift, we talked a lot about the last couple of years. Even about most intimate things, such as that Barta could not accept my soft virility and that she was looking for a new partner in order to enjoy her sexuality more intensely. Verna believed that Barta and I were going to work it out and she was there to share my needs and showed respect for my feelings. We exchanged compliments, and a spontaneous hug and a kiss confirmed our love. Over the next few days I got as far as playing her a love song over the phone on a tape recorder. We fell in love and a new chapter opened for us.

A couple of weeks later I informed Barta that I was seeing Verna whom she knew from years ago. Barta was astonished how I had managed to become involved in a new love affair even though I was so feminine. She embraced me in a final farewell. My greatest pain was that I had to leave my dear daughters; there was no chance in the future for precious relationships because their mother would not allow me to see them. Thus, I brought my two suitcases from Turbenthal to Verna's place in Winterthur. There our desires and our common ideas about life connected. Both of us had to deal with a broken marriage and without therapy we would probably even suffer from them today.

With great pleasure we decided to remarry in the cozy church above Bassersdorf in 1993. The festive mood and the congratulations of our guests gave us courage for a meaningful and dreamy beginning of our marriage. I remember Verna's elegant wedding dress, the petrol-colored skirt and bolero, her flat hat and the traditional bouquet in her hands. Her feminine shape fit the dress so well and I won't forget her cheerful expression.

We spent our time with housework, shared purchasing, walks through many cultural cities, visited clothing stores, and we always found a nice restaurant for a good dinner. But more and more I wanted my desires to be fulfilled. In 1995 I confessed to Verna that I wanted to be a woman. The time following my confession was a burden for both of us. Verna couldn't understand it after all these happy years. After all, she had married a man and not a woman, but separating would be terrible.

We kept on loving each other and thanks to an excellent marriage advisory service and therapy carried out by the Psychiatric Service of Zurich, there was hope to stay true to our wedding vows. At that time I did something without telling Verna—I went to see an endocrinologist, hoping that he would give me estrogen (female hormones) and anti-androgen (to suppress male hormones) shots. I couldn't wait to get breasts. Fat deposition around my hips and my bottom was supposed to increase, and my testicles were supposed to shrink. The doctor admired my thin body and he was very optimistic about me achieving an ideal female shape. My joy ended already after the second consulting hour. The doctor made me understand that the whole procedure would be taken over by the University Hospital Zurich. The psychiatrist looks after the patient and demands aptitude tests, the endocrinologist passes out the hormones, and the surgeon carries out the operation. Because of the delay I was disappointed, but I hoped that I'd be accepted soon. In the short term, I had my coming out and I felt liberated and happy. There were people who saw and accepted my transformation; some, though, were very surprised and thought of it as a kind of disease.

On a sunny afternoon in the spring of 1996 I went very bravely on my first walk into the city, dressed as "Armanda." I could become what I wanted with the greatest pleasure and most sensuous thoughts. I was so nervous I had to take a leak and went into a café. First I ordered the obligatory coffee-flavored ice cream and on my way back from the toilet I saw an elderly yet very neat woman sitting at my table. We made some spontaneous small talk about the waitress, contemporary fashion, and images of people, and after I had paid for my ice cream we said goodbye to each other in the most polite manner. In the mall I had the desire to buy a push-up bra and totally spontaneously an elderly saleslady helped me to find the right size. After a while in the cubicle, the saleslady asked me from behind the curtain: "Does it fit you or do you need a bigger cup?" I was lost for words, but finally I said: "It's just great, thank you." Which it was. After having bought the pretty bra, I admired my high self-esteem and thought that my feminine attitude must be pleasant to others. On my way home on the bus I knew I'd remember my first adventure all my life.

The Psychiatric Service recommended that I ought to live my transsexuality in the absence of Verna in our home, and go out in public as a woman twice a month, yet without being recognized, in order to protect the family's privacy. I like doing housework, washing, ironing, vacuuming, and pretty sewing work, which in our culture mainly is assigned to women. It is perfectly natural when I go out by car, bus, or train that I go and buy the groceries. Due to my warm charisma and my ability to communicate, I always got good feedback from all the people I met. Often I saw pregnant women, either in the company of their men or without. I felt some jealousy in my heart about them enjoying their deep love and them living their dream of having a child. Once in a park I saw a young mother on a wooden bench breastfeeding her child. Those images brought up memories of my three daughters in their youth, a very satisfying time.

My life between depression and euphoria doesn't get any rest. I'm always thinking: "Please, I want to be a woman with breasts and the female sex organs." I'm not totally against a love affair with a man, but not yet. Or with a lesbian, for that matter. According to the law, before one gets to have a sex change, one must live as a single woman for one year. In a marriage, separation is inevitable, for what woman wants to keep on having sex with a man who has undergone a sex change? In the summer of 2001 I had to see the emergency doctor. I had great pains in my shoulders and the back of my neck, but the doctor couldn't find out what the cause of this was. Yet in November of the same year, I was diagnosed with a heart problem. Consequently I had to bury my dream of having a sex change. My blood circulation was too weak to undergo an operation of many hours. I was devastated and even thought about suicide.

After a couple of weeks, I was thinking of my wife more and more; she consoled me, gave me strength and warmth. She still couldn't accept my transsexuality, but because it was impossible for me to have a sex change, the relationship gained in harmony. She has to refrain from her sexual desires, because my femininity despises the virility of the penis and the coitus.

Under the name Armanda I enjoy cultural events, especially after being diagnosed with the heart problem. I spoil myself by going to the movies, the summer theater, the ballet, country music concerts, and fashion shows. At the Expo 2002 in Yverdon, I was part of a trio of transsexuals who performed a theater show in connection with garden work. As a result, we "active women" had very thoughtful, respectful, and open-minded talks with the audience. In my free time I use my artistic talent to work on costume jewelry, brooches, or belts. I use wood, brass, and aluminum in conjunction with leather and buttons.

My pretty clothes and underwear lie in their nice fragrance in my closet. The cosmetic products in my bag and the jewelry, which carries many pleasant memories, lie in the perfumed drawers. For my feminine look I shave my legs once a month, have my manicure and pedicure done and every two years buy a short hair wig, which gives my head a youthful expression. Even Verna is very critical and honest about my new acquisitions. She likes to give me compliments or suggestions. She gives me presents, which makes my heart sing out in joy. New stockings, perfumes, clothes, underwear, earrings, and many other treasures. This makes me think that Verna looks after me like an older sister. She is very active socially and I can accept her wishes and pieces of advice gratefully. We both enjoy our shared walks, often hand in hand, loyally accompanied by our dear labrador who is very playful and willing to learn and who is always looking for our company. She shows her excitement by wagging her tail constantly. When I'm Mrs. Armanda, she accompanies me when I'm shopping or we go into the woods. She accepts my female dresses and perfumes and shows no difference in her behavior.

In the autumn of 2005 my physical symptoms got worse. I had trouble breathing and was often worn out. Since the spring of 2006 I don't work at all anymore and I get a pension. Many happy memories stay with me in my heart, and in the future I will be able to realize many joyful ideas. I'm deeply grateful to my dear wife and my kind doctors, for their competent knowledge, their advice and moral support, which enable me to live happily.

3

Our Trip to Vancouver

Jody Helfand

I woke up to the sound of the alarm. Jen was already in the bathroom putting on her makeup. She always woke up earlier than me, especially on vacations. I opened the curtains and saw an outline of trees from the window. I thought about yesterday and how we walked to Stanley Park and stopped at Lost Lagoon. We leaned over the railing and watched the ducks. One duck kept diving under the water then resurfacing a couple of feet away from where it started. As we watched it, we talked about getting married and how it would be legal here; how we could feel secure about our certificate instead of worrying about some religious freaks trying to make another amendment.

We also talked about how this vacation would be the perfect opportunity for me to touch a dick; we couldn't do this in Hawaii because it was too risky. I was already known as the teacher who changed his gender, thanks to one person, who told the wrong person, who told everyone.

The duck dived under the water again. I waited for it to reappear, but it didn't .

"I looked in the paper and found some numbers of guys we can call tonight," Jen said.

There was a big part of me that wanted to experience another man's penis; to touch it, make it hard, make it cum. I was curious because I didn't have a genetic dick. I had a two and a half inch dick without balls; one that used to be a clit.

"Let's just forget about it," I said. "We're here to get married and spend time with each other. I'll look into it when we get back."

Trans People In Love

"You'll never do it in Hawaii. You're really going to regret it if you don't leave here knowing what a dick feels like," she said, grabbing my hand.

She was right. Jen was the only person who really knew me. She understood what I needed most of the time, and she knew what to do to make sure I got it. And she was beautiful, too. Brown eyes, one lighter than the other, with a golden honey tone to it. Nice big, natural breasts; the nicest I'd ever seen in my entire life of looking at breasts. All she needed to do was touch me and I'd get hard. And it wasn't the testosterone, either. Everyone loved to blame the testosterone on every fucking thing. You're moody, you're tired, you're oversexed, it must be the hormones. But before I met her, my sex drive was definitely much lower. And the thing is that I only wanted her, nobody else, so my sex drive was always triggered by her. Her voice, her body, her touch.

"If I do this, I want you to be there," I said.

"Anything you want."

We decided to take a cab to Granville Island and walk around. The indoor market was packed, but we didn't mind. Usually we hated crowds because of the strange combinations of energy in one place, but the people here were different. They were calmer and friendlier. When I ordered my carrot apple beet juice with 1/4 apple, 1/4 beet, and the rest carrot, the person immediately understood, instead of saying, "Huh?"

We went outside and listened to a woman singing folk songs. She smiled too much and her voice was pitchy, but we didn't care. We sat on a bench and Jen unwrapped the rosemary salt bagel she bought. The air was cool and we wore sweatshirts for the first time in years. I noticed a seagull staring at us. There were signs all over Granville Island that said to watch out for seagulls, that they'll take the food right out of your hands. I reminded Jen of this and we looked at the seagull. It stared at us the way I stared at my mother when I was five and wanted a pretzel that I knew I wasn't allowed to have. I took a sip of my juice and started walking toward it, intending to give it the butter cookie I bought at a bakery in the market. I got very close to it. I could see the excitement in its eyes. I held out my hand with the butter cookie in it and the seagull took it, then flew away.

The folk singer's song ended and she started talking to the audience about global warming. Jen finished her bagel and I tossed my juice cup in the garbage. There were trash cans all over the place in Vancouver and we loved this because we always seemed to have something to throw away. We left the folk singer and walked to a huge pond. There were swans lying on the grass near the water. We sat down on another bench. I noticed a family sitting on the grass near a particularly huge swan; the child, who must have been about two, was staring at it and the mother was saying, "That's a swan. A swan. Can you say, swan?"

"What should we do for our honeymoon? It's tomorrow night and we still don't have anything planned," I said. This was so typical of us. We hated traditional things.

"Let's just stay in our room and watch some of the movies we brought with us," she replied.

"You mean like Fresh Latin Pussy #8?"

"Yeah, like Fresh Latin Pussy #8."

"Seriously, I want to do something special, something we'll remember. There must be something to do, especially because it's New Year's Eve," I said.

"#8 is definitely something we'll remember. Especially the scene where that guy takes his cock out of her ass and makes her taste it."

"That's gross."

"You love it."

"Come on, really. Let's go on a cruise or something. There must be one that leaves from Granville Island."

"I'm up for anything, as long as you follow through on what we talked about earlier."

"I don't know if I can do it. Besides, it's too expensive. Those people charge at least a hundred bucks," I said.

"You have to do this. Forget about the money. You've been talking about touching a dick for the past year and now you finally have a chance to."

She did have a point. I was pretty obsessive about it sometimes, and then other times, I'd just forget about it. Maybe because I thought it would never happen. When I started using the men's room, I would look out of a crack in my stall at the urinals to see if there were any dicks in plain view, but I could never see anything. I could hear everything, though. Especially the Ahhhhh and Ohhhhh sounds men made while pissing, but I had to use my imagination when I thought about what their dicks looked like.

"Okay, I'll do it," I said. "But I'm not getting any of his cum on me, that is if I can even make him cum. Let's go to Davie Street and see if there's anything to do tomorrow night over there."

Jen smiled and took my arm. We left the pond and walked toward the ocean. We walked onto the dock and sat down on a bench to wait for the next SeaBus. I got up to tie my shoelace and when I bent down, there was a black business card on the ground. It said "Accent Cruises" in gold letters. I wanted it to be something good, I wanted to take it as a sign from the universe that we were supposed to go on this cruise and have the time of our lives, but the card looked tacky. I put the card in my pocket and looked at Jen, who was looking right at me.

"What was that?"

"Nothing, just some business card about a cruise."

Jen put her hand in my pocket and took the card out. She looked at it for a moment and shook her head.

"Why aren't we checking this out? It looks like it could be fun."

"It's probably a huge rip-off. Besides, do you really want to be with a bunch of strangers on a cruise on our wedding day? We'll probably complain the whole time. The bathrooms will be disgusting. And we'll definitely hate the people."

"Yeah, you're right. They'll be drunk, and the food will be bad and we'll be stuck there. It's not worth taking a chance."

"But, we could go check it out just in case. Maybe we should check it out. What do you think?"

Jen smiled. "Whatever you want, baby."

Jen was good like that. Patient. She accepted my indecisiveness. She knew when my mind was made up and when I only said it was, but it really wasn't. She didn't care that I changed my mind a lot. We did have our fights, though, but many were my fault because I assumed something that wasn't true. The rest were her fault, because she assumed something that wasn't true. The good thing about Jen was that when she was wrong, she would usually admit it after a couple of hours; sometimes even a half hour. She just needed a block of time to think about the situation. I always believed that couples who didn't fight had shitty relationships anyway because that meant someone's being dishonest.

We walked away from the ocean and back up the dock to the concrete parking lot. There was a guy wearing shorts and an undershirt and that struck me as odd, because it was pretty cold out. He was leaning against a white Toyota.

"Excuse me," I said to the guy. "Have you ever heard of Accent Cruises?"

"No, sorry. Can't help you there. Can't help you. Sorry."

As we were walking away, the guy said, "Oh, Accent Cruises. Yeah, right over there."

He pointed to a floating boat and a sign that said: "Accent Cruises. New Year's, Weddings, Special Occasions. Cruise. Dinner. Dance." There was another sign underneath the bigger one that said, "Ring in 2006 In Style, From $119.95 per couple (plus GST & Dock Fee) Includes: Dinner, Noisemakers & Fireworks At Midnight."

Jen and I looked at each other and started walking in the other direction.

"That looked horrible," I said. "Don't you agree?"

"Well, it did look like a rip-off. What did they mean that fireworks are included? Everyone can watch the fireworks from a boat in the ocean," Jen said, looking back over her shoulder at the sign.

"Yeah, and we can buy our own noisemakers at a 99 cent store. I think there's one on Denman Street where we're staying."

We walked back to the dock and watched the SeaBus drive away. It was packed with passengers.

"Let's sit. The next one will be here soon," I said, sitting on the bench. "We could go to a club or we could go to Stanley Park tomorrow night. I'm sure something's happening at the park."

We were silent for a little while. I played with the zipper on my sweatshirt and she picked at her nails.

"Maybe we should just go in and see what it's all about," I said. "There's nothing to lose."

"Okay," she said. "Maybe it'll be better than we expect."

We walked back up the dock and made a right when we got to the parking lot. We walked down another dock to the entrance of the Accent Cruises' office. When we walked inside, I noticed a wall of pictures to my right. There were couples laughing, friends holding hands and hugging. And they were all on the cruise. I also noticed that there was always some type of cheap alcohol in the background.

"Hi. Can I help you?"

"We're looking for Amanda Jonas," I said. That was the name on the card I found.

"I'm Amanda."

"Hi. Well, we're getting married tomorrow and we wanted to do something really special. We were thinking about the cruise," I said.

"Congratulations on your wedding! Where are you folks from?"

"Hawaii."

"Hawaii? What are you doing here in this cold weather?"

"We hate Hawaii," Jen said. "And we love cold weather. How much is the cruise?"

I knew Jen ended with the question about the cruise so we wouldn't have to say why we hated living in Hawaii so much. We were tired of this question. Hawaii wasn't our type of place. No change of seasons, too slow a pace, and we didn't click with the scenery. We just weren't the type of people to live in a place where the sun never stops shining. And where the top story on the evening news has to do with someone's pit bull getting loose and attacking the neighbor's dog.

"The cruise costs $119.95. You get a choice of salmon or chicken, in addition to pasta, salad, bread, coffee, tea, and dessert. That price also includes a bottle of champagne. We have pictures on the wall over there if you want to see what it looks like."

"Is there still space left or is it filling up fast?"

"It's filling up pretty fast, but there's still some space left."

"We'll have to think about it," I said, knowing Jen would agree.

"Thanks for stopping in. I'll be here for another hour and we accept all major credit cards, checks, and cash," Amanda said.

We walked outside. "Should we do it?"

"I think I'll leave this one up to you," Jen said.

"What if it sucks?"

"It won't suck because we'll be together. And we could always make fun of the people and the music if it's really bad."

We walked back inside. I got out my credit card and gave it to Amanda, who booked us on the New Year's Cruise. "Your reservations are confirmed. Be here at 6:00 p.m. to board. Have fun, you two. And congratulations again on your wedding!"

We decided to skip Davie Street and took a cab to English Bay to watch the sunset. We sat on the grass and watched two dogs playing with each other; one was gigantic and the other was half its size, but they played well together. I held Jen's hand and kissed her neck. Her skin always felt so soft on my lips. I decided to bite her shoulder.

"Ouch. That hurt," she said.

"But did it feel good, too?"

"Yes."

"Let's forget the dick thing tonight. We can do it the day after the wedding. I'd rather be alone with you."

"This better not be a trick. You're going to touch a dick before we leave Vancouver. Promise me."

"Okay, I promise, sweetheart."

Jen loved it when I called her sweetheart because it sounded old-fashioned. She also loved when I called her sweetpea because when she was younger she fantasized about meeting someone who would call her that. When I said, "I love you, sweetpea," about five months into our relationship, she was shocked, because she never thought she would meet someone who would call her that. And then after about eight months into our relationship I did something else she had always wanted a guy to do—I took her face in both of my hands and kissed her. After that, she was hooked for life. It's hard to admit, because some would say it's sexist, but after I saw her tits, I was hooked for life. That was only one week into our relationship. When I seriously think about it, though, it wasn't only her tits; it was everything. The way she kissed me, the way it felt when she touched me, the way I felt when I touched her. The way we could talk about anything and not feel uncomfortable. The way she peed on my couch when I made her laugh too hard. When that happened, my first instinct was to just clean it up. It was no big deal to me. Actually, now that I think about it, that must have been after I fell in love with her, because if she were anyone else, I would have gotten rid of the couch and bought a new one.

We continued walking until we reached Denman Street. There were too many people near us. They were walking too fast and speaking a variety of different languages. One person spoke French. Another spoke Japanese. Another, Spanish. I liked the multicultural aspect, but I didn't like the feeling of claustrophobia I was having. Then some guy's arm brushed against mine.

"That's it," I said. I gotta get out of here. Let's go to Hornby and Robson. The woman at our hotel said there were some good restaurants around that area."

"Good idea, I'm starting to get cold. Let's get a cab."

Five minutes later, we were warm inside a cab on our way to Hornby Street. Ten minutes after that, we were sitting in Bellagios, a restaurant the cab driver recommended. The waitress came over to our table and gave us our menus.

"I'll be with you in a moment," she said, smiling.

"I like our waitress," I said.

"Me, too."

Liking the waitress was important because it meant that our meal would taste better. Every time we went out to eat, we always decided whether or not we liked our server at the beginning of the meal. If we did, it put us in a good mood. I put my napkin on my lap and looked around. The hostess seated us in a booth in the corner, away from people. The light in the restaurant came mostly from lamps and the walls were painted a deep red color that was almost maroon. There was a painting above our table of a violin and in the background there was a garden with roses and tulips.

I stared at Jen from across the table. "You're so beautiful," I said.

Jen always thought I told her she was beautiful to make her feel good, but that wasn't true. I told her she was beautiful, because she was. And I wasn't the only one who noticed. When we went places, I saw guys looking at her. I didn't like it, but it happens when you're with someone who's hot. When I'd tell her about some guy who looked at her, she'd say I imagined it and that there were always girls looking at me. If they looked, I didn't notice or care. The fact was, I was in love, and most of the things said about love were true; I only have eyes for you, you're my one and only true love, all those sayings I thought were bullshit were actually true. I just didn't know it until I met Jen.

"So are you nervous about tomorrow?" Jen asked. "Did you write your vows?"

"Why would I be nervous? Yeah, I'm nervous. I didn't write them yet. Don't rush me, these things take time. Did you write yours?"

"This morning, when you were sleeping. Did I snore last night?"

"If you did, you didn't keep me up."

The waitress came back and we ordered our food. Then she said, "Do you mind if I ask you both something?"

Jen and I shook our heads. "No," I said.

"How long have you been a couple?"

"Almost two years," Jen said.

"Why do you ask?" I said.

"Well, I couldn't help but notice how engrossed you two were in your conversation. I mean, I put your drinks and the bread down earlier, and you guys didn't even notice. It was like I wasn't even there. You were in your own world. I see a lot of couples come and go, but most of them don't have the connection you two have. It's nice to see it. Very refreshing."

"Our souls are connected," I said.

"It's obvious."

"It didn't come easy. At first, everyone disapproved of our age difference," Jen said.

"You have an age difference? I never would have known."

"Yeah, fourteen years, but we're the average of our ages, which makes us both twenty-seven," I smiled and the waitress smiled back.

"Are you married?"

"We're getting married tomorrow," I said.

"Really? Congratulations. You guys are a really cool couple. I'll be back," she said, and walked away.

"Do you think she's straight, bi, or gay?" Jen said.

"Definitely straight."

"I think she's a lesbian."

"Let's ask her."

"No way, are you crazy?"

"I'll ask," I said.

"No, please don't. Don't ask, okay? I'm asking you nicely."

Jen got embarrassed easily sometimes in front of strangers. I never got embarrassed in front of strangers. I could fart, burp, talk loudly about unpleasant things, cuss, etc. and I would never care about what anyone was thinking. But I toned it down a little because I didn't want Jen to feel uncomfortable.

"Okay, I promise. I won't ask."

Jen came and sat with me on my side of the booth. "Thanks, husband."

"Do you believe that we'll have the same rights as everyone else and we'll be recognized as a married couple? It's pretty surreal," I said, putting my arm around her shoulders.

"It wouldn't be if we were born in Vancouver," Jen squeezed my thigh and went back to her side of the booth.

We stared at each other for a couple of minutes and listened to the music that was playing. The waitress came back with our food.

"Calamari and maple salmon, really really well done. Check the fish and make sure it's okay."

I took the salmon apart with my fork and it was cooked completely. "Perfect," I said.

"My partner is just like you. She likes her fish really cooked. Raw fish freaks her out."

Jen smiled at me. The expression on her face said, I-told-you-she-was-a-lesbian. Then she looked at the waitress. "In Hawaii, raw fish is pretty popular, but we don't eat it."

"It's popular here, too," the waitress said.

After the meal, the waitress put the check on the table. "Let me know if you want anything else. I hope I see you two again. If I don't, have a wonderful day tomorrow."

"Thanks," I said.

I looked at the bill. "Could this be right?" I handed Jen the check.

"I knew she was going to do that," Jen said.

She only charged us for the drinks. I left a twenty dollar bill on the table with the check and we got up to go. It was dark by the time we were finished and the air was crisp.

"It feels so good out here," Jen said, grabbing my arm. "Do you want to get a cab or do you want to walk back?"

"Let's walk."

We made a right on Robson and walked toward our hotel, passing some souvenir stores.

"Let's buy a t-shirt for Danny," Jen said.

We walked into a store and picked out a cute little blue shirt with a whale on it that said "Vancouver." "Will 4T be too big for him," I asked.

"He'll grow into it," she said, walking over to the magnets.

I thought about Danny for a minute. He was Jen's son. She had him when she was still in high school. She told me she used to hide in the bathroom in a stall during lunchtime and that the kids at school called her a slut. But she only slept with one guy and they were both virgins when they met. When he found out she was pregnant, he left her for another girl. Everyone told her to give the baby up for adoption and she agreed to, but six months into the pregnancy she changed her mind because of a dream she had. She was sitting in a rocking chair holding a newborn baby. Her grandmother, who recently passed away, walked over to her and said, "This is a special baby and you have to keep him." She woke up knowing two things: That her baby was a boy and that she would keep him.

When I found out about Danny, I didn't mind. I never really liked kids, but I knew I'd like hers because she was part of him. He was almost one when I met him, and he didn't turn away from me and ignore me the way he did with other people. Instead, he stared at me with extreme curiosity. It was like he knew I would be in his life for a long time. Sometimes I would rub his back in his crib after he woke up crying. He always fell asleep within minutes and I was shocked at how fast my touch soothed him.

We left the shop and Jen grabbed my hand. "I'm craving your cock," she said.

"It wants you." I squeezed her hand.

We passed a natural foods store and an internet café. In a couple of blocks, we'd be back at the Times Square Suites. We'd sit by the fireplace and kiss. Then we'd move to the bed and have amazing sex.

* * *

I felt a hand on my shoulder. "What are you doing standing there by the window? Did you write your vows yet? We have to leave in an hour and you haven't even showered or eaten."

I turned around. "I was just thinking about last night."

"Mmmmm," she said. "Wanna do it again later as a married couple?"

"What do you think? Now leave me alone. I have to write my vows."

I continued to look at the trees. I waited for some kind of inspiration, but it didn't happen. I sat on the bed and opened my notebook. I wrote a couple of stupid things down like "I love you, I'll always love your ass," and then ripped out the pages and tore them up.

I didn't know what to write. I didn't know how to tell her that I'll always work for our happiness. That I'll never stop loving her. That I'll be with her for the rest of my life. That I'll never leave her.

I looked at the trees again. I remembered a line from one of my favorite poems: "But the place endures." I thought about the trees. I wrote the line down and stared at it. I continued writing until I was finished. I read it out loud to make sure it flowed and then I ripped it out of the notebook and folded it in half, and then half again.

"Okay, I'm finished," I yelled.

A minute later, Jen came into the room. She was wearing the red dress we bought at Nordstroms that showed off her curves.

"You look incredible," I said, putting my arms around her.

"Stop it."

"You look incredible," I said again.

"You just like the way my tits look in this dress."

"You better believe it. They're my tits. I own them!"

"Mmmm hmmm. Now get that hot little ass in the shower before you're late to your own wedding."

I walked into the bathroom and took off my clothes. For a moment I stared at my chest in the mirror. Then I turned on the water and waited for it to get hot.

4

To Fight, Live, and Love
at the Gender Border

Isaac Lindstrom

It was me
It was you
I am your black triangle
You are my red circle
I have sharp edges
You are soft and round
I am stone
You are the sun
I penetrated you
You embraced me
I was dark
You gave me some light
I was in heaven
You let me be there
You and me together were no longer two separate signs but
    one single symbol of love.

(In this poem and in the following story I am referring to the butch-femme symbol created by Daddy Rhon. Thanks for a wonderful and powerful symbol of passion and love).

Trans People In Love

A PRESENTATION FROM THE GENDER BORDER

This story is about a person who doesn't feel comfortable with the sex assigned at birth, a person who fights wars with the body almost every single day, a person who fights for being seen as the transgender stone butch man he identifies himself as, a person who struggles for recognition, a person who seeks to be accepted and recognizable in this world, a person who loves to learn and who feels very comfortable at a university, a person who is a foreign adoptee, a person who lives in Sweden, a person who fights, lives, and loves at the gender border—this person, I suppose, is me.

My gender identity is male. Outside the gay, lesbian, bi, trans, intersex, and queer (GLBTIQ)-context, in other words, in the rest of society, I identify simply as a male or as an FTM. Inside the GLBTIQ-context I identify as a transgender stone butch man. I haven't yet taken any testosterone or done any surgery but I live full time as a guy, at the university and in the streets. I hope to start taking hormones and to have top surgery done in the near future.

I often describe myself in terms of colors to make people understand. If pink and blue represents a girl and a boy, I am turquoise. This color is a rather appropriate description of my gender because people often argue over whether turquoise is blue or green. It is a color that is hard to easily define. I just want to explain what I mean by that metaphor. I am a guy but not an "ordinary" (what is ordinary?) guy. Not that I don't want to be an "ordinary" man but I don't think it is a possibility for me because I will always, for good and bad, carry with me the experiences of being given the wrong sex at birth and living (or after transition having lived) in a body that doesn't feel like it's mine. And even if or when I go through a transition (which I am hopefully planning to do, at least some parts of it) my body will not be exactly the same as if I was born with a male body.

I don't think we ever will be able to find some genuine gender core or say things like, "You have XX-chromosomes and therefore your essence is that of a woman" or, "You don't like wearing a dress and you want to have a beard and therefore your essence is that of a man." It's all formed by language and discourses about sex and gender. The language is set out in front of the "I," comes before the "I" and constitutes the "I." In some ways you are not the owner of your own words. What I am saying is not that I deny the possibilities of an existing gender core but that there isn't a clearly defined point in which you know what gender you are. That doesn't mean you don't have experiences and feelings about being the sex you identify with but it means that your experiences are formed by language. That is not to claim that your feelings and experiences are worth less. They are as real as any experiences can be.

Okay, maybe you are wondering why on earth I bother to go through taking testosterone and having surgery done if sex isn't something essential. Well, that's hard to answer briefly, but first of all it is because of the slow-moving nature of discourses on gender and secondly because every subject (even the transgendered subject) is always within the discourses. There is no standpoint from outside, no pre-discursive domain from where you can speak because your speech is already a discursive one. It means that I am too as a transgendered person in the hegemonic discourses of sex and gender. I too as a transgendered person "know" what a female and a male is.

If you want me to express my sexuality in terms of homo-, hetero-, or bisexual I am definitely a monogamous heterosexual man but I prefer to say that I am femme-sexual or simply that women turn me on. My sexual preference is absolutely for femme women and the more feminine the better. That doesn't mean I am unable to love other people. That fact is I don't think love and sexual passion must go hand in hand.

EXPERIENCES AND THOUGHTS FROM A STONE BUTCH

Now that you know at least a little about whom you have in front of you, I want to share with you some of my experiences, thoughts, and reflections about being a transgender stone butch and in love. The problems, the possibilities, and the attractions. I also want to share some thoughts about being stone and the pleasures and problems with femme partners. I will also share some of my thoughts and experience of having a relationship that lacks a word to signify it, and I'll tell you about my hopes for the future.

I am not in a relationship right now, so what I'll give you are glimpses of my past experiences. I have chosen to talk about single events organized into the following themes:

- About being in love: a princess kissed my heart
- About being loved: when she wants a me that isn't me if you ask me
- About being stone
- About my feelings when the two signs become one symbol
- Love and sexual attraction are by default not necessarily interconnected
- The future

So you don't know exactly what I have done with whom, I've omitted people's names because I don't want to give anyone away.

About Being in Love: A Princess Kissed My Heart

After a long conversation and flirting on the Net, when I first met you in real life I thought you were an angel or a fairytale queen. Your hair was extremely long and blonde and you were wearing something that to me looked like a pink princess dress. You had the most perfectly formed lips painted in pink. They looked like a heart wanting to be kissed. Indeed I ached to kiss that heart.

My brown and your blue eyes met for the first time before we embraced each other ever so gently. You smelled sweet like a wild rose and your skin touching mine felt soft against my skin. Oh, my knees went weak and I had butterflies in my stomach. The only femme in the world was you. You really caught my interest at first sight.

We left the crowded school yard and went to a nearby café. I drank my black coffee and you sipped on your café latte with sugar. People went by and I felt so very proud being there with the most wonderful femme ever. I looked at your sweet hands and fantasized about them stroking my neck.

When we were finished at the café we walked side by side along the road. It was a perfect warm summer's day with a blue sky and not a single cloud. We chatted about everything and nothing. I really don't remember what we talked about because it wasn't the oral talk that spoke to me. No, it was your eyes in mine and your smiling pink, perfect lips and the sound of your crystal voice.

We went down to the water and found a silent bench under a huge green tree. A dog barking from far away was the only sound except for you and me breathing. The sun was already on its way down and it painted the sky in orange, red, and purple. You sat next to me. Your dress was short enough to reveal your legs. You sat with one perfect leg across the other perfect leg. You said you thought I was very handsome and that the shirt and tie I was wearing were so romantic, like a handsome butch in a dream. I felt my cheeks getting hot and I slowly reached for your hand and kissed it.

The evening turned into night and the summer sky was now filled with shining stars over our heads. The warmth of the day was all gone and we both felt the cold wind. I gave you my black leather jacket to keep you warm when we walked back along the road the same way we came. We walked the road hand in hand this time. With my princess by my side I was the happiest transgender stone butch in the whole world.

We stopped. I kissed your perfect lips and I really wanted to come deep inside you in all sorts of ways. You ran your fingernails along my neck and I was shivering with pleasure. I sighed. I was in love with you and never wanted this moment to end, but it did.

Well, my thoughts about you being a princess haven't gone away. I still think you are a princess, a princess of all transgender stone butches' hearts.

About Being Loved: When She Wants a Me That Isn't Me if You Ask Me

The music was very loud and the dance floor was crowded with people jumping and bumping all over. The red, blue, and yellow lights formed circles, stars, flowers, and triangles on the floor and on the walls. The air was dense with smoke. I walked across the dance floor from the bar to some tables. I was pretty tired after a long day's work at the university. I sat down next to a woman and took some sips from my Guinness. We looked at each other and I could see in her eyes that she found me interesting. We talked but the noisy music was too loud so I missed a lot of the conversation. Well, never mind.

We did some dating and had a nice time together even if I can see in retrospect that we both pushed the limits and tested each other. That's absolutely not a healthy relationship. I want a woman to be a woman and she wanted me to be a woman too, (yuk!); yes a butch, but still a woman. She wanted me to be something that I can't be and I wanted her to be something that she couldn't be. The problems really kicked in when it came to sex. It felt good when I was in charge, when I was the one who fucked her. The problem was that she didn't always want to be passive. She wanted me naked and she wanted to do to me what I did to her and of course it just didn't work out.

I admit that I knew from the beginning that this wouldn't work but I couldn't imagine how bad it would turn out in the end. At first I thought it was okay with her not to give and for me to be the one who was always on top of her. She wasn't exactly my type and I think I wasn't hers either, but stupid me was on her anyway. What I am saying is that there's nothing wrong with her. Absolutely not. She is a wonderful person but the combination of her and me was all wrong. You live and learn from your mistakes, that's for sure. At least I hope so.

About Being Stone

Imagine having parts of your body that you don't feel at all comfortable with because they don't feel like yours. When you look at yourself in the mirror you see a body that has parts which belong to— what you and the rest of civilization has learned is a she— but you are a he, not a she. Do you want anyone to touch, focus on, and desire these body parts that you feel so terribly wrong about? Well, maybe you do and there's nothing wrong with that, but I don't.

The problem according to me is that all bodies are sexed, and what sex a body is or has (is sex something someone is or something someone has?) is regulated through a binary gender scheme which categorizes sexed bodies according to rigid gender norms. Therefore, we don't have any access to refer to a pure body and I have my doubts that such a body even exists. The body is always a discursively produced body.

What I want to express by stating that I am stone is at least two things. First and foremost it says something about how I am in the sheets and how I am as a partner. It is not possible to touch parts of me that aren't a part of me or want me to be undressed. If she doesn't understand that if she desires things I don't have, then she doesn't love the man I am, but a she. I am not a she and therefore she and I are just not a good idea. If she says that it should be all right to touch me and that she can imagine that it is a male chest or if she says to me that my body is all right just as it is, I don't think we will work out. If she thinks I am anything else but the active dominant part in bed, she is totally wrong. I am not a switch. I am the one in charge and the one who does her, not the other way around. If she thinks there should be no penetration at all, no domination, just mutuality, I respect that, but well, what boring vanilla. No thanks! I think she would do better as my friend than as my woman.

Secondly the word stone signifies that I am a person who is pretty hard to get near or to get to know. But the people who are inside the border really have a great friend to trust for good times and bad. I have experienced both—when she couldn't cope with me being stone and when she liked it, and expressed that it was exactly what turned her on and that she didn't want me any other way.

When a woman identifies as a lesbian my experience is that it seems to be hard for her to desire me the way I want to be desired which is not strange at all. If she is a woman who only feels attraction to other women, and I am a he and she desires me as a she, the whole thing easily results in two frustrated and misunderstood people. No good for any of us. I don't want her to be interested in parts of my body that I "don't have." I don't even want her to fantasize about them. To ask me to get undressed or to ask to touch "the nonexisting" parts is horrible. I have a butch-cock and that's what I want to use and what I want her to fantasize about. I want her to look at me as a he. That's why I now try to avoid lesbians.

It also seems to be a bit hard, at least before my hormones and surgery, for straight women to find me attractive. After I take hormones and have surgery if a straight woman does find me attractive, and if I find her attractive too, what on earth should I then do if she doesn't know that I was assigned another sex at birth? When should I tell her? In the beginning? I don't think I am able to keep it secret when it comes to sex (like in *Boys Don't Cry*) even if sometimes I wish I could. Well, I have to think this situation over so I will be prepared for this day. This really is an issue for me because I am pretty sure this day will come.

I remember one time when I had a night out I danced and talked to a woman without her knowing I am transgendered. She looked at me as a he and wow, it felt just perfect! Even when we danced very close she didn't think of me as being anything other than a he. I never told her. Why should I risk ruining the evening? I must admit that if a straight woman should find me attractive I would feel just perfect because her desire is for a he and that's the way I see myself and want to be recognized.

Once a bisexual woman told me that she thought I was attractive. In the end she hurt me but she gave me the most wonderful words to keep, when she said that she wanted me as her edgy black triangle. She said she couldn't see me as anything else but a he and that my butch-cock is no less real than any other cock. She wanted me by her side as her man and she wanted to be my woman. She was so feminine, both in appearance and in the way she acted and talked. She said that she felt attraction and passion for me, and wanted me to wear my leather jacket when we were having sex. She didn't want me to take any of my clothes off. She said she felt fine with being the one who was pushed against the wall, laid down or flipped over and penetrated. There was never any talk about whether I could do it the other way around and to switch was never even an issue. She wanted to be my red circle; round, soft, and shining. She said she wanted the black triangle to always stay within the red circle so that it felt the love and warmth that would never leave.

What a joke! She said she was the monogamous type but after a while I realized she was dating not one but several other people at once. Shit! Why do I always have to share my woman with others? That's something I will not accept! Am I not worth more than that? "Yes, I am," I say to myself, trying to build my self-esteem (It's hard to love yourself when you all too often have to confront the fact that things are wrong about you). My dream was ruined yet another time. I felt hopeless, fooled, and angry. I thought like I sometimes do that my life would be easier if I just managed to control or turn off my lust and my sex drive. But how? What a wonderful sweet dream it was, she and I, before everything got ruined. Why does a dream like that seem to be so hard to keep?

About My Feelings When the Two Signs Become One Symbol

A black triangle and a red circle. Just two different colors and two simple geometric forms. So plain and so simple but in its simplicity it forms a powerful expression about passion and love. Not primarily about sex but about the few perfect moments when I feel in harmony, when I don't feel like a stranger in this world, like an object not fully recognizable. Those moments when I can be the man I am without being questioned by both myself and by others. For a short period of time my being just feels natural. (I usually don't like to use the words natural or being but when it comes to this I am willing to make an exception to the rule.) This is when the two simple signs become one great unified symbol in the act of healing and rebirth.

You may think it silly to talk about a sex act in religious terms but for me this is almost like a religious experience. Therefore, I now want to share one of my memories from last year. It was late autumn and I was away for a few days on a seminary listening to the Anglican Bishop John Shelby Spong. At the end of the seminary I got to swap a few words with him, just me and him. I told him that his theology brings hope to transgendered persons like me and that I have a hard time with, not necessarily God, but the church, the Bible, and the hard Christian dogmas like Jesus who died for our sins, the virgin Mary, and the story of creation. He embraced me and said (I cite from memory): "You have all the potential to be what you are meant to be and remember that God will always love you." Despite the fact that I consider myself very influenced by post-structuralism and by the thoughts of Judith Butler—Butler's theories about subversive performativity, materialization, and so on is helping me a lot in my struggle for creating a, as Butler puts it, liveable life and I am so very grateful to Professor Butler!—there were some tears in my eyes and I felt a little hope starting to grow in my chest.

Why am I telling you about some words from an Anglican bishop? This text shouldn't be about God but about love, shouldn't it? But you see, the words from Bishop Spong were right on the mark to explain the glimpses of eternity in the love act, glimpses when I can be just someone who is.

Like in the poem at the beginning of the text, the black triangle is both penetrating and at the same time embraced. The edge deep down in the red circle and in its center explodes with pleasure. The sun lightens up some of the darkness in the act of healing; healing of wounds inflicted by the experiences of being an object in the world. When I look into her eyes and feel in all of her open trembling body that she desires me and when she moves with me like in a dance of harmony, then I am in heaven. For that single moment I am what I was meant to be (to refer to Spong's words). For in that single moment I am a man who is and the love welcomes me home.

Love and Sexual Attraction Are By Default Not Necessarily Interconnected

Why do some people have such a hard time understanding that some of us are perfectly capable of separating sex from love or love from sex? There is nothing wrong in feeling love, romance, and sexual attraction for the same person. No, what I am saying is that people (like me) who sometimes can and do separate these two, have the same right to feel what we feel without being looked at with suspicion.

As you know, the only thing that turns me on and awakens my sexual lust is feminine women. That doesn't exclude others like butches, men, lesbians, or any other people to become someone I love and have near my heart. I can even have romantic feelings for people other than feminine women, but not sexual lust.

At the time of this writing my nearest and most beloved person is a bisexual Bear man. I have known him for five years now and I hope there'll be more years to come. I really do love him and he really loves me. I love him in a nonsexual way. As far as I know a word doesn't exist to describe our relationship and that's one of the problems. How do you easily refer to a person with whom you have a nonrecognizable relationship? We are more than friends but we are not a couple and it is not a sexual relationship. The ancient Greeks sometimes talked about a man loving another man without sexual feelings between them and I think maybe they meant such a kind of love as he and I have. When I am in trouble or feeling down he is the one who is there for me. When I am happy and want to share my happiness he is there for me too. When he is in trouble or feeling down I am the one who is there for him. When he is happy I am the one to share his happiness. We also share intellectually with each other. We read and comment on each other's essays and it's just wonderful to sit for a whole day discussing post-structuralism or queer theory with him.

I love to sit next to him, hold his hand, and watch the sun going down over a red and orange sea. I love to look at his bearded face and to look in his kindly blue eyes and feel our souls connected to one another in love and trust. I love listening to when we both are singing and our voices meet to build a beautiful and strong harmony. I love when we do weird things like driving around in the middle of the night and stop outside a church at the countryside to eat hamburgers and French fries. I hope nothing in the world will ever come between us and that I will have him near my heart and he will have me near his, even when I get old and time is running out.

The Future

What are my hopes and wishes for the future? Well, as I told you in the beginning I have a great passion for books and for university. My wish is to continue the journey and to dig deeper into that world of theories and reflections.

My body? Hopefully I'll soon start a journey, a journey on shaky black water and silky white sand. The journey is a hard one but it's the only choice I have. It's the only way for me to make a home in this world. It's my struggle for a liveable life and I have a battery of theories with me, helping me to interpret the relation between the "I" and the world and I am still picking up more. I think I know my destination well. Maybe it's just an illusion but it can't be. What is illusion and what is reality? What is true and what is false? Those stupid dichotomies! What is an I? What is a true man? What is a real cock? What makes me less of a man than someone who was given that sex at birth? I don't know the answers. You don't know the answers either because the true answers aren't out there to be found on an ontological level.

I have many thoughts and wishes for the future about how my body will change when I am on testosterone and when I have had my top surgery done. I feel a little nervous about the result. I know that the changes take a long time but I can't help wanting it to happen overnight. But I have the patience to wait and one of the important things is that with hormones I will grow old as the correct sex, not as a woman, but as a man. What a wonderful future to have a body that is at least the most mine can ever be. It will also make it easier for a future partner to see the me that I identify as me.

About my wishes concerning a woman? I also told you that I am a monogamous, heterosexual, femme/woman-loving man, so what I hope for is to find a healthy long-term relationship. When I say long-term I mean long. I want the whole thing. I hope some day to get married to a beautiful, feminine, monogamous, faithful woman who calls me her beloved husband and I'll call her my beloved wife. I can imagine the fantastic feeling when the priest pronounces the words, "You are now husband (wow, it's really me!) and wife." I hope to find a woman who sees me and who wants to share both living and loving.

What about children? I am really not the type who likes children. I have never, ever been able to think about myself as a mother. It makes me sick! I remember an episode when I was about eight years old and someone asked me whether I wanted to become a mother when I grew up. I screamed "NO!" She just looked at me and patted me on my little head and said, "You will change your mind when you become older." I was so upset, angry, and frustrated. I thought that she didn't know what she was talking about and that she was all wrong. She had not the faintest idea that she was talking with a transgendered person. Even the faintest thought of being pregnant makes my guts turn inside out with pain and agony because it isn't me! It has always felt terribly wrong.

When I instead started to think about being a father, things changed and it's now extremely clear to me that if I am going to be a parent at all in the future I must be a father; anything else is absurd. Something that bothers me, though, is that I will never be able to get my wife pregnant, no matter how much we make love. But I can be a father anyway. Science gives me and my future wife lots of opportunities. It is ethics that creates the limits. The future will tell if I feel grown up enough to become a father some day, though I do have my doubts.

Two things at least are certain. I really want to be a damn good husband to my woman (if she comes my way some day) and I always want my platonic love to be near my heart.

5

Perfect Day

Susan Stryker

I still think of it as my perfect day; some day whose date I can't remember now, in June 1980. I was a few weeks shy of my nineteenth birthday and had blown every last cent of my savings to get myself to Europe, to spend the summer back-packing around to "find myself." For the first time in my life I was entirely outside the contexts of family and friends, away from everybody who had any expectations of who I was or what I was supposed to be.

I'd made it across Germany and France to the UK and had worked my way north from London to the Lake District, when my perfect day arrived. I was staying at a hostel in Ambleside, and had planned a day of ridge-walking—just me in my woolly gray sweater, low stone walls, contented sheep, and stunning views. I had been unwinding for weeks, visiting places I remembered from my army-brat childhood in Bavaria, getting my first taste of Paris hauteur, thrashing in the moshpit at Hammersmith Palais when Burning Spear opened for The Clash. I had been to Stonehenge and Stratford-on-Avon, and now I was setting off to commune with the souls of romantic poets, a slim volume of Coleridge tucked in my day-pack. I look back fondly, with some bemusement, on how sincere and naive I was then.

My thoughts were drifting, as teenage thoughts are wont to do, and turned to the question of love. I had been dissatisfied, I had to admit, but I myself was largely to blame. I had not been honest with my girl-friends—all four of them at that point—about what I was really looking for in a relationship. It was impossible to separate what I wanted from them, from what I wanted for myself.

Trans People In Love

I can't honestly say that I considered myself a lesbian at that point in my life. I was born male, but had puzzled over gender as long as I could remember. Gender had never been an assumption for me, but had always been a question. When I was very little I remember nonchalantly thinking, that I would grow up to be a woman. I'm agnostic about where these thoughts and feelings came from, but they were phenomenologically persistent and undeniably real. When I realized, around age five, the normative relationship between genital difference and social gender, it surprised and shocked me. This presented a *huge* problem. Were my self-perceptions wrong? Had I made a mistake? Or was everybody else wrong about me? What was real, and what wasn't? Who got to say who was a boy and who was a girl? Why, I wondered, did the pronoun "she" feel like the one I wanted to name me? Why, when somebody said "he" in reference to me, did I shrug inwardly, with the unvoiced qualifier, "Well, I understand why you might think so, but that's not really what I am?" These early conundrums became the bedrock of my later intellectual life, as I pursued an unlikely career as a transgender theorist, historian, and filmmaker.

Living as a boy was nonconsensual. I had been plopped, never asked, into a gender I would not have chosen. I accepted my status only provisionally, pending further assessment of my situation. I didn't know if it would be possible for me to leave, any more than if it would be possible for me to stay. I started dreaming of bodily transformation as a potential escape route. I dreamed of machines that changed the shape of my genitals, gave me breasts, made my hair long. I dreamed the emotional logic of coercive normalization within consumer capitalism: some adult would recognize my girlish proclivities, take me out to buy girl things but then laugh at me, as if they had successfully pulled a prank, when I admitted that I really thought of myself as a girl. I would always awaken feeling furious and betrayed.

I turned bookish, always looking from the corner of my eye for answers to the gender questions, and became precociously erudite in the process. My mind was often elsewhere than my body; still, I didn't let the unresolved status of my gender identity paralyze me. I tried to get on with things and make the best of it. I didn't needlessly resist my socialization, picked my battles, bided my time. I watched war movies, played football, swam competitively, learned to swear like a motherfucker, and get stupid in public with alcohol. Like everybody else, I learned where the boundaries were drawn between masculinity and femininity, and knew where I was situated. I learned that voicing questions about gender did not elicit helpful answers, and sometimes created problems for oneself. Truth be told, I always felt like being a guy was a perfectly fine way of being in the world. I was just never convinced it was *my* way. I wondered why it mattered what gender you happened to be, but still couldn't shake my sense of preference.

I dreamed about girls, starting around age six. It usually went something like this. A classmate or neighbor-girl I thought was really funny or smart or cute or nice would confess she had a secret crush on me. (A black-haired, dark-eyed tomboy beauty in my first-grade class, who showed up at school every so often looking uncomfortable in a pink Jackie-O skirt and suit jacket, was my first such inamorata.) My family, however, would be on the verge of moving away (which we did with some regularity in real life). The girl would want me stay with her, and her parents would agree to take me in. All of my clothes and toys would accidentally be sent away with my own family, and then, due to some emergency like falling in a mud puddle or being attacked by a stray dog, my only remaining set of boy's things would be ruined. Of course, my girlfriend would lend me some of her clothes until mine could be replaced, whereupon she would then discover, much to her surprise and delight, what a nice little girl I made. Her parents would be accommodating; they'd always wanted to raise another girl, and my own parents miraculously agreed to let me stay. She and I would be friends—not boyfriend and girlfriend, just friends, practically sisters. We would do all sorts of things together because we really liked being with each other, and would be best friends forever. Somewhere around puberty, these dreams became sexual. What could possibly be sweeter than discovering that your best friend, who you shared so many special things with, *loved you,* in a special sort of way?

So I wasn't quite a transsexual lesbian, on that perfect day in the Lake District, a few weeks shy of my nineteenth birthday in the summer of 1980, but I was pretty darn close. I just didn't know what to call myself yet.

Somewhere between the ages of ten and thirteen (based on where I remember living at the time), I read a *Dear Abby* advice column in the newspaper. A woman wrote to say that she had discovered her husband had been sneaking into her closet and trying on her clothes; she wondered if her husband were secretly homosexual. Abby told her that homosexuals were people who loved people of their own sex, and that it didn't have anything to do with cross-dressing. She said the woman's husband could possibly be a transsexual, who was a person who considered himself or herself a member of the opposite sex, but that most likely her husband was a transvestite, who was somebody who had no desire to change sex but enjoyed wearing the clothing of the opposite sex. Eureka! Language is truly a gift from the gods. Not only did I now have definitive proof that I was not the only person to have ever questioned their own gender, I also had a vocabulary to help me frame my thoughts. And off to the public library I rode, unconsciously fey, on my purple Schwinn Sting-Ray with the banana seat and sissy bar, handle bar streamers flying furiously in the wind.

The library was hugely disappointing. "Transsexualism" was indeed listed in the subject classifications of the card catalog, but the only books treating the topic were textbooks of abnormal psychology. I read that transsexuals were deeply disturbed people who feared being homosexual, or who felt guilty about being homosexual, and who wanted to be members of the other sex so that their sexual feelings would appear normal. Sadly, I concluded that I was not a transsexual after all, because not only did I not consider myself abnormal, I also did not consider homosexuality repulsive. In fact, I thought it sounded pretty cool. My own budding desires revolved around what the porn magazines stashed under the mattresses in friends' bedrooms called "girl-on-girl action." I knew that if *I* was one of those women in the magazines, I wouldn't gingerly touch the tip of my tongue to the tip of hers, or place one long painted nail against her nipple—I'd crush her lips to mine and fondle her breast voraciously as she fondled mine. What I didn't know was how to put my body into the stories I saw in those pictures, or into the fantasies of transformation I dreamed of at night.

I decided that, since I obviously wasn't transsexual, I must be some heretofore unnamed kind of creature. In retrospect, it seems like it would have been so easy to put two of those terms I found together, to name my emerging sense of self as both transsexual and homosexual, but at the time the categories seemed mutually exclusive, so round and round I went: I feel like I'm really a girl so I *could* be transsexual, but if I'm transsexual I'm supposed to want to be with guys, but if I'm transsexual in order to be with guys then that means I'm repulsed by homosexuality, but I'm actually attracted to homosexuality, especially homosexuality in women, but a homosexual woman wouldn't like me because I have a guy body, but I could be homosexually involved with women if I were a woman, and I could be a woman if I was transsexual, but I can't be transsexual because that means I'm attracted to guys and repulsed by homosexuality … and in the end, teenage passions being what teenage passions are, it was easier to just keep my mouth shut and date the women who wanted to date me, all of whom happened to be straight.

And that's what I was thinking about as I walked along the ridge lines of the Lakeland Fells, on my perfect day. I was wondering who I would love, and who would love me, and how we would love, given the complexities of my gender. My girlfriends had all been nice people, and I still carry happy thoughts of good times with them all. One was a fiery-tempered cheerleader running away from an abusive father and living with an older brother. Another was a sweet, pot-smoking rock-and-roll groupie who was one of the most relaxed, fun-loving people I've ever yet encountered. The third was a high-strung, mixed-up daughter of nouveau riche parents; she had—I kid you not—two uteri. For the fourth, I was a way of rebelling against a controlling and overprotective mother. I enjoyed sex with them all. It actually felt fantastic to penetrate their vaginas with my penis, because it felt like my penis had gone away. It wasn't dangling about and poking around, but was put away someplace nice that let me push the little spot at the base of my shaft that I always thought of as my clit right up against my girlfriend's bush, and grind against her until we both came. While fucking, my penis—superfluous——disappeared.

All my girlfriends thought I was such a sweet boy, said I wasn't like the other guys, said they could talk to me, said they liked the way I listened to them, said they appreciated that I liked to do things with them besides fuck, and seemed to enjoy my just hanging out with them. Then something would happen, some slip, some anti-gay slur, perhaps. Maybe they would laugh the wrong way when television comedian Flip Wilson did his "Geraldine" character, or make gagging noises when talking about transsexual tennis player Renée Richards, whose story was then much-covered in the daily papers. It was always something, some little pin to burst the bubble of what she and I could, in my dreams, be to each other. I would know then that she was not the one for me. Not that I ever let on, until the usual vagaries of time drifted us apart.

It wasn't much of a climax, my little epiphany, that afternoon on the ridge. It was more like something dropped away. I had been shedding bits of my familiar self for weeks, all across Europe, when another little piece of scale fell from my inner eye, and I found myself alone at last in a quiet moment of clarity and insight. It simply became obvious to me that I would never have a meaningful relationship with a woman unless I told her how I really felt about myself, which was that I loved women, had a male body, had never thought of myself as a man, didn't seem to qualify as a transsexual, and had never been turned on by anything other than the thought of being in a lesbian relationship. The question of whether or not I would ever try to change my body, if that was somehow possible for a normal nontranssexual like me, or what kind of body I would have, or how I would live in public, had to be an open-ended question within the relationship. I didn't know yet what kind of flaming creature I was, but I wanted companionship while I tried to figure it out. I wanted to find somebody who was interested in the process. I decided that, upon returning home, I would make a point of dating bisexual women—women who knew how to eroticize a relationship with a woman but could enjoy making love with a male body. I would come out to my lovers about my sense of self early in the relationship, because if they couldn't hang with the situation, it was all for the best that things end quickly. And that, a few weeks later, is precisely what I did.

She was in my fencing class. There was something about the way she sat cross-legged, her unapologetic armpit hair, her awkward brashness, that big sexy Jewish nose that tipped me off. Dyke. Probably a hardcore feminist. I was smitten. Not being properly socialized into the subtleties of womyn-loving-womyn courtship, I tried to engage her with some stupid conversational gambit, and if she hadn't noticed that I was left-handed, she probably would have blown me off and life would have been very different. But left-handers have a slight advantage in fencing—our attacks always come from the off-side in relation to most everybody else—and she wanted to practice against me. We spent the next decade fencing with each other, and we both drew blood in the end.

I loved that she would engage with me, fight with me, play with me, argue with me, take me as seriously as I took her. I loved that she spoke German. I loved that she loved movies, and would talk about them and not just watch them and eat her popcorn and be done with it. We would disagree passionately over why we both liked the same thing. Our first date was a triple feature of Bergman, Fassbinder, and Herzog. Our second date was *The Rocky Horror Picture Show.* By our third date we'd come out to each other—she wasn't sure she liked guys, I wasn't sure I was one. It worked for both of us, more or less, from the time I was nineteen until I was almost thirty. We got married, went off to graduate school together, made a home together, had a child together. I was so happy being seen through my lover's eyes. I thought I knew what the shape of my life would look like. But I was wrong.

There was that nagging little question about my embodiment. We circled around it. All of our sex fantasies and bedroom stories and erotica-reading were lesbocentric. All of our family life felt gender-egalitarian—how we split up the chores, how we parented, how we took turns with work and school and supported each other. It felt like lesbian domesticity. I grew increasingly disenchanted with only my lover seeing me as I saw myself. The person I was to myself, the person I was with her, was not the person I was to everyone else who mattered in my life. She insisted that I keep the matter between us alone. I grew increasingly alienated from my genitals, but was perfectly happy to fuck with fingers, tongues, toys, or anything else. By this time, I'd come around to the conclusion that, regardless of what some old textbooks had said, one could in fact be a transsexual lesbian; that one had the power to name oneself. It was just a matter of persuading others to go along with you. I started describing myself to my partner as a preoperative transsexual lesbian who was still living as a man but no longer wanted to do so.

She did not want me to change. She feared what her family would think. We had both read feminist and lesbian literature and knew the feminist party line on transsexual lesbianism—no fake females allowed in the club. She feared we would be ostracized, would have no community, wouldn't find work, wouldn't have a place to live, would be poor and marginalized, our parents would disown us and our child would be scarred for life by the stigma. These were not unrealistic fears, and she wanted to be safe. She wanted to retain heterosexual privilege, even if she felt she was queer. My body was her closet, and she didn't want me to come out.

Things turned ugly, in all the ways that divorce is usually ugly. One afternoon, after a sleepless night filled with bitter grief and mutual re-criminations, I was lying, dazed and spent, in the grass beside our apartment building. I felt as if my entire life was being ripped away, and the void was staring into me. My thoughts spun back to that per-fect day, a decade earlier, when familiar life had been stripped away in a more pleasant fashion, and I consciously stepped onto the path that led me here. I found again, unbidden as before, that same sense of inner clarity that welled within me then. The path went forward. I took my step, she and I parted ways, and I started my transition.

Regrets, I've had a few, but not about transitioning. Regardless of how it might have affected my relationships with other people, it's what was right for me. Nobody else can live my life for me, so how I live in my body for myself is the necessary basis for every other rela-tionship I have with anyone else. I'm completely clear about that now. Fortunately, all of the people who really mattered in my life, ex-cept my ex, stayed with me through my transition, and I found won-derful new people along the way to share life's adventures.

I started living as a woman in the early 1990s in San Francisco, just as "queer" (as opposed to old-school baby-boomer gay and lesbian) was coming into currency. I'd never seen a good place for myself in the old economy of sexual identities anyway, and felt very comfort-able calling myself queer. I was gender queer. I also liked a new word that started getting tossed around about this time, "transgender." I felt it fit me, and created a bit of distance between the old medical mindset associated with "transsexual" and the bohemian life I was living. I cared nothing about passing, everything about being seen for what I was: a queer woman in the process of leaving a male body be-hind. I didn't care, if my girlfriend didn't, that I still sported nonstan-dard equipment. I was saving my pennies to replace the factory in-stalled model with something custom-built anyway, and just wanted her to love me and have crazy, sexy fun while I scraped my surgery money together. I wanted her to look forward to the prospect of eating me out as much as I looked forward to spreading my legs for her.

Life, in many respects, became a dream come true. My body, and the life I lived through it, was finally aligned with the structure of my deepest desires and identifications. I was happy. I had been prepared for a solitary existence post-transition, but found that I was desirable to many women I desired. Lesbian transphobia, while real, turned out to be more monolithic in theory than in practice. I went wild for a few years, dated widely, played around casually, frequented orgies, slept my way across town. No names, but a few college professors, a couple of magazine editors, a stripper, a secretary, a dominatrix, a tattooist, a performance artist, a lawyer, a graphic designer, an abortion clinic manager, and two butch dykes in the process of transitioning female-to-male. (If I've forgotten anyone, forgive me.) I learned to see myself in relation to a lot of different women (and a few men), and I came into my own.

I would have been content to live my life with three of those people. One was dating someone else at the same time she was dating me, and ultimately chose to be with the other woman. I was sad, but these things happen, and I got over it. She and I run into each other now and then at professional meetings, and sometimes get together for a drink when we happen to be in the same city. I always think it's nice to see her. Another I would have shacked up with quite happily had she felt able to leave a long-term nonmonogamous relationship. We had horrible timing with each other for years, one of us was involved in a primary relationship with somebody else when the other was free, and vice versa. After a while, we reconciled to the fact that for each of us the other was "the one that got away," and we settled down into a really warm, close, and ongoing friendship. The third became my life partner throughout my thirties.

She was younger than me by eight years, punky butch-of-center in appearance but an outdoorsy granola dyke just beneath the skin, same shoe size as me and almost my height, with hazel eyes like my father. We lived a life we considered self-consciously radical: polyamorous, collectivist, anarchist, activist, artistic, intellectual. I didn't have a regular job and made my living teaching around as adjunct faculty, writing books and magazine pieces, picking up speaking gigs, doing odd jobs and piece work, while doing my part to turn transgender studies into a recognized academic field. I told people I was just a girl who lived by her wits, and it was true. It was hard economically, but it was also utterly, romantically, wonderfully, free—just another word for nothin' left to lose. We felt like we were reinventing the world, reinventing family, reinventing love, reinventing ourselves. She had a child we co-parented, along with my son, and we lived with people who felt more like kin than roommates. We all somehow managed to buy a house together before the dot-com boom drove real estate prices through the roof. It was a big place, and we turned it into a commune. We had the best dinner parties and the most interesting houseguests in the world. Somewhere along the way I finally had my surgery. We thought we were the revolution. And in a way, we were.

Revolutions have a way of turning out other than you expect, and this one was no exception. Our former housemates partnered up and moved away, and we started renting out rooms. My partner started her own business, started writing books of her own, and that took up a lot of her time. I landed a postdoctoral fellowship, and then accepted a job as the executive director of a nonprofit organization. I worked a lot. The kids were getting older, and just schlepping them to school and karate and play-dates with friends took a big chunk out of the daily schedule. Life wasn't quite as wild as it once was, but I felt fine. I felt like I was turning into the woman I'd once imagined I'd grow up to be.

Maybe it was lesbian bed-death. Maybe it was, truth be told, that she was freaked out by my genital surgery and it triggered her survivor-of-sexual assault issues. Maybe she had been too young when we got together, and she had the best of intentions but just grew in a different direction. Maybe she never loved me the way that I loved her. Maybe it's that she secretly wanted to be monogamous. Maybe it's just that she fell in love with somebody else. Maybe it was that I'd gotten fat, or liked to drink more than she did, or would sometimes self-medicate my stress with nicotine. It was probably all of the above. After ten years that felt to me like our relationship was getting steadily better, she suddenly bugged out and left me for one of my former students, a trans guy I'd tried to mentor, somebody as much younger than her as she was than me. It blindsided and shattered me. For the second time in my life I felt like my world had crashed, but this time there was no salving memory of a quiet inner place, unexpectedly encountered on a perfect summer day. There was only pain.

That was five years ago, but what they say is true—time is a healer. I'm in a new relationship now and so far, so good. My current partner is somebody I had dated during my polyamorous days with my second long-term lover, so she'd already been in my life for some time. After my unexpected breakup we saw no reason to stop seeing each other, and we moved cautiously ahead. A year or so of inconsolable grieving on my part, tentative steps toward new couplehood, weekly relationship counseling (we are, after all, middle-aged, middle-class lesbians, for whom psychotherapy is a subcultural norm), and finally moving in together about a year ago. It feels solid. It feels like we've both been around the block a time or two now, and know how to do relationships right this time. We take nothing for granted.

It's not always easy between us, but it's mostly the routine kind of not easy. We both have kids from previous relationships with us part-time, and blending families is sometimes a challenge. There are some unresolved in-law issues. We're from different class backgrounds. She's detail-oriented and I'm a big-picture gal who's fuzzy on the small stuff, which sometimes creates tension. She pouts when I travel, and I get annoyed when she kvetches. We both like to get our way, and usually think we're right about everything. Some nights, one of us winds up sleeping alone in a huff. She'd been a lesbian for twenty years before she met me, but now that we're together some of her old friends have distanced themselves. I'm sorry that she's suffered a loss for loving me. We've made new friends together, though, and kept the best of her old bunch, as well as mine. My crowd thinks she's swell.

So, where does that leave us? We love each other and try to be nice to each other, because life's too short for unnecessary unpleasantness. We like traveling together, and watching movies at home. We've established a good domestic rhythm. We find each other sexy. She often laughs at my jokes and I think her smile is exquisitely beautiful every time I see it. We take pleasure in our work, and our material needs are abundantly met. We enjoy our hot tub and a cold cosmopolitan cocktail on chilly San Francisco nights. Sometimes when I'm soaking, watching the low clouds scuttle in from the sea, I think back to that perfect day, the summer I turned nineteen. I came down from the ridge in the evening, and walked back into town, where I picked up some lamb meat, rosemary, and potatoes to make myself a stew. After dinner I drew a hot bath, and threw open the big leaded glass bathroom window to look up at the hills I'd climbed earlier in the day. The steam rose and the water cooled as I lay in the tub, and the dusk turned darker and the nighttime fell. I look at my partner and think: I have a lot of perfect days now.

6

A Transgressor's Love

Andrés Ignacio Rivera Duarte

It's not easy to be a transsexual man, every single day hating a body that doesn't belong to you, hating every period, hating those breasts stuck on your chest that you're forced to see day after day, feeling them in the shower and binding them tight so that no one else can see them. And it means knowing how people make fun of you, treating you like a faggot, a lesbian, a tomboy, or calling you any other name just to offend, humiliate, and discriminate. Accepting your body and soul, accepting yourself just the way you are . . . maybe this is something strange, maybe it's freakish.

When the psychologist told me in my thirties that I was transsexual, I thought that I had to be the only one. How could there be anyone else like me? What kind of celestial mistake was I? Why this punishment? Would I ever be happy? Would I ever find a woman who could love me? Would I ever enjoy walking on the street wearing a shirt and tie? What would my family say? My father, mother, and brothers are so close to God, to the Church; they are believers and go to Sunday Mass; they teach the catechism—they're the perfect Chilean family.

I couldn't face it. I preferred to be a coward and keep quiet rather than face my family. So I lived the deceitful life of a professional woman who at home was a man. I kept to myself and remained a nobody. I stopped socializing, going to birthday parties, dinners, and movies. In short, I became a hermit with every year of this living death marking a step closer to the end while I hated every centimeter of my body.

When I was thirty-eight my father got cancer and I decided to be with him during his last months. For the first time ever, we talked

Trans People In Love

about life and its pains, frustrations and mistakes, but we never talked about how different I was. On February 27, 2002 my father passed away in my arms. Feeling his last breath touched my heart and mind; I faced death and realized that shutting myself away was destroying my life. In the same year I had a mastectomy, without telling my family anything, but after a time my mother realized, and when she reproached me about my life, I confessed to her that I was a transsexual man.

My mother erupted in hatred and became a different person; she spat blood and fire from her eyes and mouth and searched for any words that could hurt me more and more. But finally I realized that I had to live my life, I couldn't keep on living just for society, for my family, fearing what other people might say. I needed to become Andrés, and I needed to live him intensely.

I used to hang out and talk with my friend Inés, who helped me through my transformation. One day she invited me to meet two of her friends at a restaurant. Inés and I arrived together, and before we entered, my eyes wandered to a table inside where a pair of blue eyes lit up a beautiful face. It was Inés's friend, and knowing that we would soon meet, I got nervous. I was a transsexual man, dressed in male clothes, still in the closet; she was beautiful and so feminine.

Finally we locked gazes and our cheeks brushed against each other in a "hello" kiss that moved my heart so strongly that I thought it might jump out of my chest. I sat down to share a soft drink, and we talked and laughed. I made the offer to take her home so I would have a chance to find out where she lived, even though we ended up going with Inés, but we left open the possibility that we might get together again. After she left, I immediately told Inés that her friend was beautiful and that she had to arrange for us to get together again. Her eyes had touched me so deeply and her lips had begged me to taste their delicious flavor of love.

Two days went by and we saw each other again. We barely realized how quickly the time was passing, and we started to become friends. We started seeing each other more often and we had so much in common. She had wounds of the heart just like me. She had a violent and failed marriage that left her with two children. I was a transsexual man only just now starting his life. She was twenty-nine years old with two children, aged five and six, and I was thirty-nine. She gave off an air of sensitivity and I was hurt and cranky. She had a sensual feminine essence while I was sometimes shy and quiet.

One day she was telling me about the failure of her marriage and she started crying so I hugged her. What a feeling! Even today, I can remember it and my heart beats faster . . . feeling her body next to mine, her breathing on my chest, the fragrance of her hair, softness of her hand touching my arm, feeling her so close to me and her body fitting my body so perfectly. I soothed her pain, cradling her in my arms until her tears no longer wet my shirt. I wiped her face with my handkerchief as she thanked me with a sweet look of grateful comfort. I didn't kiss her and she didn't kiss me but for both of us the feeling of that comforting hug remained. When I drove her home we didn't talk much. I was totally wrapped up in remembering every second that I held her in my arms while she was looking out through the car window.

Two months after the day I was first bewitched by her eyes, by her mouth, it was time for me to tell her that I was a transsexual man. I didn't know how she was going to react, but I knew I had to be honest. I invited her to go out to the countryside where nature's landscape could amaze us with its flowers and trees. As I drove I told her the truth. A deep moment of silence followed until she looked at me very calmly and said, "It's not your body I care about, it's *you,* you're special. And I think I have a special son, too, and you help me understand both of you." Then she hugged me and I cried in her arms. For the first time I felt accepted for what I am inside, not for my body, so that I too might feel comforted and respected. I felt her warm arms and chest, where her breasts rose against my face as she breathed. It was an endless embrace that finally closed with a kiss on the cheek that told us we were friends.

The days were going by and we saw each other more and more often. We started needing each other, sharing, laughing at my three-month-old puppy's crazy games. We recorded and listened to music, enjoyed the outdoors, a dewdrop sliding down a rose petal, a cup of coffee, or a glass of wine.

One afternoon we were sitting on the floor with our backs against the bed, and my dog was playing around, running, jumping, biting my ear, and pulling my hair. He just wouldn't let us talk quietly. To keep him from biting me I moved dangerously close to my love's face. It was just for an instant, a second that we looked at each other. We were breathing fast … but we moved apart without saying a word, silently concealing behind a smile what we felt, watching my dog play.

She was alone that day, without the kids, and she didn't want to spend the night alone. I told her she could stay with me and that we could sleep together but that she could trust me to be respectful. She looked at me and decided to stay. I found her some pajamas and while she was changing in the bathroom I got all sweaty and nervous. I was going to have her in my bed close to my body. I'd be able to feel her essence with every breath, maybe hug her, smell her hair next to my face. There were so many thoughts and feelings at that moment.

Finally she was right next to me, lying down, and I smelled her fragrance. We talked and looked at each other, and then she said she was tired and turned over to go to sleep. At that point she snuggled with her back against my chest and I put my arm around her and pulled her closer. I don't know how long we stayed like that but I think it was a long time. I started to caress her arms going slowly up toward her face. My kisses traced her outline, eyebrows, cheeks, chin, and lips. Those perfect lips —so perfect—the lips of a perfect heart asking for me to kiss them.

Her mouth parted. Slowly I turned her toward me and kissed her full on the mouth with my tongue playing with the shape of those beautiful lips. My hand explored every centimeter of her body. Then I moved closer to her belly, brushing against her breasts hoping for some response. It came with a tender kiss that built to a full passionate one. My hands were on her breasts. Her nipples were so hard and her breathing became full of excitement. My lips were moving down her neck, kissing it, biting it, moving lower until my lips found her nipples. I kissed them. My tongue played with them as I got on top of her, pressing my belly against hers. Then my hand came down to her vagina and I felt her nectar moistening my fingers. I went down with my lips to feel her nectar in my mouth, her juices in my mouth feeling the contractions of her clitoris as I kissed and caressed it with my tongue.

I felt her excited breathing, her breasts heaving up with every breath; I felt the wildness of her legs, her moans of ecstasy and pleasure. I drank in the explosion of her nectar with every detail filling my soul with happiness and my life with a new light. Looking at her face, seeing those eyes and lips transported me along a path of flowers where each one flashed and shone its colors. Although there was so much fear in her eyes, hands, body; so much fear of the unknown—a transsexual man with a vagina and a clitoris. I softly embraced her and whispered that we would go slowly, overcoming every obstacle along the way and that making love is also about enjoying the nectar of our union. There was no reason to hurry, she would relax, take her time and feel comfortable caressing me and experiencing me as much more than just a person with a vagina.

Morning found us still entwined in bed, and we looked at each other shyly and kissed. We knew that something had been born and that we were committed to each other. She went home carrying my heart away with her. At that moment I understood that she was the woman I wanted to grow old with. Hers were the eyes I wanted to see just before mine closed forever. Hers were the hands I wanted to hold as we walked through life together. Hers was the fragrance I wanted to smell next to me every morning and every night; and that it was her nectar I wanted to drink every day to nourish me with feminine tenderness and passion. After a few hours I went to her house giving her chocolates as she looked at me tenderly. I just gave her the chocolates and whispered in her ear, "Thanks for letting me be happy," and then I left.

The next day we got together again and when we saw each other the passion naturally flowed. Again, every single centimeter of her body was caressed by my lips and tongue as her clothes fell from her down to the floor. The passion came often as we grew closer together. I talked many times with my partner about the way we were growing and bonding. We discussed her initial fears and doubts about being with a man who had a woman's body. She confessed to me that at the beginning it was like having all the wires crossed in her brain. She's heterosexual, used to be married, and likes men. Then she met me, liked me, started needing me, valuing our conversations, laughter, and playing. Her thoughts were that if I were not there she would feel all alone. She started questioning her feelings as to how she reacted to our intimacy, to our mutual gaze and laughter and felt that her body wanted to be closer to mine. The desire inside her rose and in spite of my woman's body, she saw, felt, and loved a man—Andrés Rivera— the man I am.

As the days went by I got to know her children, sharing, playing, and going out with them. They started to see me as part of their life as we spent time as a couple, which developed into a family. After two years we told the children that I'm a transsexual man and an activist because I was going to be on television. The children with their natural directness and wisdom asked many questions and we were prepared for them, having taken the advice of a psychiatrist about how to face that moment. Today they are nine and ten years old and also take part in social activism. We've included them in some activities and they've gotten to know lesbians, gays, transsexual men and women, all in a very natural way. They know what discrimination is and they're going to teach society about respect.

Four years have now gone by since I saw my partner for the first time but her eyes still light up my heart with infinite love that has cured my pain. My breath quickens just to see her, my chest swells when I hug her, and when my hands caress her body I see my own reflection in her eyes. We are still together building a family without our parents or siblings, who, frightened by the weight of moralistic social opinions, distanced themselves from us after my public coming out. In my partner's case, her family doubts the relationship, the love and the genuineness of our feelings; failing to understand that love has no gender or sex, that love lives and breathes in a person without needing a name, and that love simply comes to us so that we can nurture it and live it.

This loving path has emerged over my transsexual journey of a hysterectomy, hormonal treatment, the growth of my clitoris, the broadening of my back, the deepness of my voice, the growth of hair on my face, back, legs, and belly, the replacement of feminine characteristics by masculine ones, integration into society, work, activism, and the struggle for human rights and equality.

Through this transformation I became myself. I showed myself in public as a man, standing up to everyone including my family. Yes, I can now fight for equality and fairness against great odds. I became an activist, the president of the Transsexual Organization for the Dignity of Diversity in Rancagua, Chile. I accept the duty of sensitively and intelligently educating people about these issues by speaking before school and university groups and other organizations.

Today I lead my life as Andrés Rivera, an activist, in love with a wonderful woman with whom I've built a family based on honesty where the children know that I'm a transsexual man. Their mother is also an activist who shares my fight for equality and freedom from discrimination. She is a brave woman who is not afraid of what people might say. This is a woman who stays by my side, lighting up my life with her wonderful eyes and feeding my soul with her nectar and kisses.

This road hasn't been easy. I have suffered rejection, humiliation, and discrimination from my family. My brothers are publicly ashamed of me and won't let me see their children. Society rejected me and I was unemployed for two years, which led to depression and alcoholism, and one time I tried to kill myself. But I also had the strength to dream. I dreamed that we could build a better world, a fairer and more equal world, and my dream gave me the strength to stand up and become an activist and it moves me forward today. My dream also allowed me to build myself as a man so that I could walk alongside the woman who has sheltered me with her love and healed my pain with her kisses but most of all helped love grow inside my soul.

7

I'm Not a Lesbian, My Wife Is: Norms and Perceptions in a Trans Marriage

Gypsey Teague

I met my future wife, Marla, at a religious convention that I was hosting in 1994. Religion like gender, however, is often a misnomer, and this conference was such a venue. There at a small and very conservative hotel in Amarillo, Texas over 200 pagans and witches gathered to celebrate the fall. We had Wiccans, Norse, Dianics, Gardnerians, Georgians, and a scattering of the more eclectic paths, all in one hotel for one weekend.

Marla had come with her high priestess and was new to this particular convention. We were both coming out of bad divorces, and ironically, had both asked the Goddess to bring someone into our lives, with Marla going as far as to ask for someone who wouldn't make her life boring. It goes to exemplify the adage "be careful what you wish for, for you just might get it."

At that time in our lives we were both sexually adventurous. I had just started, and quickly ended, a relationship with a very attractive guy and Marla was enjoying being single after a long marriage. We were also both perfectly suited for each other in the mainstream of society, she being genetically and physically female and I being genetically and physically male. We began dating that night and have been together ever since.

I feel some background at this point may be in order. From the time I was a senior in high school I have been involved in one form or another with the transgender community. The brother of a close friend of mine transitioned that year and committed suicide just after my

Trans People In Love

graduation from high school, due to family and community pressures. In 1970, being transgender was equal to being insane or worse and s/he couldn't handle what society was dishing out. Ironically, out of my graduation class from high school we had a number of pressure-related suicides, one from a 4.0 student the week before he was to leave for Harvard. Whether coincidence or divine guidance, from that moment on I have had contact with the community through personal friendships, business, social, or outreach services. Interestingly enough, though, is the fact that I never wished to be female, never felt the urge to cross-dress, even at Halloween, and didn't fully understand the drive to align identity with form. I was just cognizant of the needs of the individuals on a very simplistic level.

Shortly after getting married, Marla and I opened a clothing boutique in Norman, Oklahoma and began selling gowns, shoes, erotic leather, and high-end toys for the more risqué. To sell these items more efficiently to the fetish and bondage, domination, and sadomasochism (BDSM) communities, and to make money in secondary sales, we began doing fashion and drag shows, showcasing our wares, and donating the money to the state AIDS hospice. As the owner of the shop, I was called upon to MC the shows and began doing them in drag, just as a lark. I also sang and camped around on stage during the fashion portion, but never as a way of life, although at that time I had the ability to switch from the male mode that I lived in to a fully female mindset within seconds and once in drag was both acceptable and passable as a woman.

In 2000 my father died of what we thought at first was asbestos poisoning but later learned was testicular cancer. Shortly after that I was told by specialists that I had the same fate looming ahead of me, unless I did something drastic, due to a military vasectomy that had produced large amounts of scar tissue around the testicles. That something drastic came in the form of estrogen therapy, much like the therapy used for prostate cancer survivors today. You get high doses of estrogen to shrink certain tissues to preclude the metastasization of the skin and tissue.

I accepted this short-term therapy with pragmatism and began taking Premarin. I was on that drug for six months when my medication was changed to delestrogen, Prometrium, and spironolactone. Every six months I would get a new dosage and a new prognosis. After two years I began encountering hot flashes, crying, night sweats, and so on. It was not something that I had ever experienced when younger and it was quite unpleasant at times. Usually late at night when Marla and I would talk about our future and what might happen if the therapy didn't work, I'd get emotional, start to cry, and then sweat a wet spot in the bed. It was a hard year to say the least.

To this point my story was pretty similar to a million other transgenders: hormone therapy, even though for an unrelated reason, go through the first two years of transition, again for an unrelated reason than most, and begin to show the effects of that therapy; larger breasts, wider hips, softer skin, less body hair. None of these things bothered me since I expected to have them disappear once I was off the hormones.

I was also going to a therapist at Marla's suggestion. All my life I had been less than thrilled with life. I've been a military officer, martial arts black belt, mountain climber, scuba diver, and a hundred other death-defying sports and vocations but none of them really excited me. She, therefore, thought I was depressed and had me find someone to talk to. After six months of therapy the clinician said I was not depressed, just not happy. When I pressed him for the difference he said he could prescribe something for depression. As for being happy, he said I was on my own.

During this time I was a library branch director at the Historic Black University in Oklahoma, and teaching marketing and management at the campus. On a Friday night, during the spring semester of 2003 I was giving a lecture to my capstone management class when one of my male students said something very male and very sexist. I vividly remember saying, "You don't understand. You can get a raise because you can pee standing up." I then caught myself before I said "we" and said, "The girls have to work twice as hard for half the pay." It was then that I realized I had just self-identified with the women in the class. Within a month I had lost the ability to think of myself as male.

Shortly after that, Marla was talking to a friend of hers online and the friend mentioned that she was transgender and her mother had been prescribed DES (diethylstilbestrol) for miscarriage when she was pregnant with her. My mother had also had miscarriages before having me and I investigated to discover if I too was a DES baby. Over the next six months, slowly becoming more female in my identity, while holding out that I would be off the hormones soon, I found that DES affects the brains of unborn males, keeping them from imprinting male, thus 25 percent of DES baby boys are born with female brains. As a child I never suffered from that feeling of disconnection that many other transgender people cite, but now I was feeling alienated from my own body, a body that was changing with or without my approval.

Eventually the hormones in my system reached a "toxic" level, so to speak, and an irreversible tipping point occurred where my female brain overwrote my male brain. My therapist assured me it was quite possible to do this and also quite irreversible. At about the same time, I began passing as female, again nothing that I either anticipated or desired.

Let me give you a few examples and then a few more of how Marla reacted to them. The first time was in the Oklahoma City airport while waiting for my flight to a conference. I was in a t-shirt, jeans, sandals, with my hair about to my ear lobes and brushed back. I had no make-up, nail polish, or jewelry on, nor was I trying to act feminine. I simply had to pee. As they called the first boarding to my flight I walked into the men's room. There in the entryway a large gentleman barred my way and said, "Jesus lady, this is the men's room." As my flight boarded and he refused to move, I had two options. Pee on his leg, thus missing my flight altogether and dealing with security or going into the ladies room, which I did—I sat down, peed, and got on with my day. I think I was in too much of a hurry to think of the ramifications of my actions so I hurried in, finished, and hurried out. I laughed to myself as I got on the plane because for a couple of years prior I would always angst over which bathroom to use when I was out and about in drag, between shows, or in other cities and dressed. Now, here I was, fully dressed as male and using the ladies room with no problems. It should be this simple all the time.

On the way back through Dallas I stopped for Chinese food at the concourse and the second odd thing happened. Without looking up, the man behind the counter asked what I wanted and called me "Sir." When he looked up at me he smiled and said, "I'm sorry ma'am, what may I do for you?" Again, I was taken aback, but recovered, ordered, and paid for my food with a "Thank you ma'am," from the cashier.

I told Marla what had happened and she said they were flukes. She was about to find out just how wrong she was. We took my mom out to get her nails done at Wal-Mart. While she was there I went over to get a new pair of jeans, since my hip gain made the ones I owned fit badly. I asked the lady at the changing area for a pair of black dress jeans. Without hesitation she pointed to the women's section and said, "We have White Stag, Rider, and Lady Wranglers." I settled on a pair of black Riders and came back with one pair to try on. Trying to be a good boy, I said "one" and took the ticket toward the men's side to my right. The woman stopped me and said, "We're on this side here, hon. You're thinking of the other store," meaning the other Wal-Mart had the women's changing rooms on the right.

This continued every time we went out, almost from that moment on. Once while wearing a necktie and button-down shirt I went with Marla for lunch at the mall and the hostess asked, "Would you ladies like smoking or nonsmoking?" That was the beginning of months of slowly being squeezed out of the male part of society and into the female portion. Within a few months of those incidents there were very few places, other than work and home that would even deign to think of me as male.

Also at that time, our relationship began to change. Marla began to wonder if she could or wanted to be perceived as a lesbian. I was becoming someone that she loved, yet someone that she didn't marry nor expected when we met. I don't believe the anger had begun yet, but there was concern in each of us that these changes, some looking like they'd be long-term, were going to happen, with or without our approval.

Finally with the physical changes, the change in self-identity, and the knowledge that I would never get off the hormones I was taking, Marla and I talked about genital reassignment surgery. We set a date for real-life experience to begin, cleared it with my therapists and gynecologist, and then I met with the campus director.

A little history of the university system in Oklahoma seems in order. It is almost impossible to sue a state university, and even harder to sue the black university in the state. Also, at least on the campus I was at, discrimination was alive and prevalent. The pecking order was black males, white males, black females, white females, and then others, to include Hispanic, Asian, Native American, and finally transgenders on the bottom. After meeting with the director, though, he assured me there would be no problem with transition and I would be treated with dignity and respect. First lie.

I next met with the associate vice president of the entire university. She also assured me that I would be treated as a trusted member of the faculty and that no discrimination or prejudice would be tolerated. Second lie. Lastly I met with my students that I supported as a library director and professor and they also said they would support me in my transition. Third and final lie.

Through all of this Marla and I stuck together. At first we expected the situation to improve, and when it didn't, we were already so bonded emotionally, spiritually, and physically, that the physical problems were not as insurmountable as with many other couples going through similar situations. That was fortunate because when it started going bad at work she was the only normalcy I had.

The first incident was when I had been living full time as a woman for a month. I came back from a conference where I was a presenter to find over 100 hate letters about me being transgender all over the campus and my library. To add insult to injury they were signed and dated by the student distributing them and they were copied on campus staff equipment. When I asked the director of the campus for some support I was told the student could say whatever he wished and that the director would not get involved. After my attorney contacted the main campus I received an audience with the associate vice president, who repeated the campus director's sentiments. I could not seek redress against the university since the state would not approve a lawsuit; the students had the right to say whatever they wished about me, and the administration was there to support the students over the faculty.

At the same time, I was told to use the faculty bathrooms at the other end of the building, even though all the other faculty members used the student bathrooms across from my library. When I brought up the other faculty members' use of student bathrooms I was told that there was nothing the administration could do about the other faculty members but they could do something about me.

During this time I chose to have surgery to remove any chances of falling victim to what killed my father, and I interviewed at Clemson University, with their full knowledge that I was transgender. The surgery was successful and so was the interview. I was offered a job at Clemson to start in May of 2005 as the branch head of the architecture library. I did not tell my home university about the job, though, because when I got back from the interview I found a death threat had been circulated through the building, saying that in the name of God I should be removed. The implication of that statement was quite evident. Again no help from the university. Their only action was to tell me they were changing my teaching schedule starting the next semester from 5-7.30 p.m. to 7.30-10 p.m., knowing that the branch campus was in the darkest, most crime-ridden section of Oklahoma City and that I would be the only class that would meet those nights.

Thirty days from my start date at Clemson, and with thirty days of leave built up I gave my notice in Oklahoma. They had a week to deal with me leaving, which is probably what kept me safe, since it was too quick to do anything to me, even spontaneously. Marla helped me move to Clemson, South Carolina on May 1, 2005, and I cried all the way back to my new apartment when she boarded a plane to fly home to Oklahoma. At that time I thought it was the beginning of the end of nine years of marriage. Marla was dealing with the emotional implications of me as a woman and if she would be satisfied living as a lesbian

The distance and separation only made us more convinced we were meant to be together. Within six months, Marla found a position as the Director of a Technical College library five miles from Clemson and moved to South Carolina. From a heterosexual couple in Oklahoma to a lesbian couple in South Carolina, we adjusted. Where most stories would end, this one just started. As a male librarian with multiple graduate degrees I was just another voice in the crowd in Oklahoma. However, once I arrived at Clemson I found that I was the only male-to-female transgender faculty member at a state university in South Carolina. Add to that the fact that the president of the university had just put into effect a nondiscrimination policy that included sexual orientation and I became a much sought-after speaker and asset.

Ironically the week I received my death threat invoking God's wrath in Oklahoma City, I was given a plaque for being one of the outstanding researchers at the same university on the main campus. The plaque was for my work on the evolution of gender thought, which was published in a peer reviewed journal, and for my editorship of *The New Goddess: Transgender Women in the Twenty-First Century.* Now at Clemson, *The New Goddess* was published, and everyone wanted me to speak about being a transgender in South Carolina. I found myself giving interviews, doing radio shows, giving packed auditorium lectures, and being the guest speaker at classes, and seminars throughout the state. I joined the women's studies department as a faculty member and began developing and teaching gender and transgender courses for undergraduate and graduate credit.

Once Marla moved to South Carolina, and explained our situation to those she worked with, we settled into a normal life as a perceived lesbian couple. We bought a house in a cute little development that already had one lesbian couple up the street, joined the Unitarian Church, and their welcoming committee for GLBT parishioners, and made friends in a community where sexual orientation and past body parts are not an issue. On the surface, living in South Carolina was a great improvement to Oklahoma.

But not everything is what it seems. True, Marla and I go about our daily lives as two women, living together, but the climate is still hateful to lesbians and gays. Just this year a state amendment was passed making marriage restricted to one man and one woman. The irony is that even though the state of South Carolina, the federal government, and the state of New Hampshire all agree that I should have an F for female on my documents, Marla and I still have a valid, heterosexual marriage license from Oklahoma, where we were originally married as one man and one woman. Further, and this may some day have to go to court if pressed, genetics are still on my side for the marriage issue. I am, and always will be, genetically male, as are all my transgender sisters worldwide. Nothing will ever change that, so if pressed, we are still legally married, genetically.

The most challenging part of living as two women together has not been the distribution of domestic chores; we both cook equally well, and are both very neat and orderly women. Nor has it been the fact that we are both clothes collectors, a cost of doing business in a profession where you are expected to look better than average. It is the physicality. I have always been attracted to women, so becoming one did nothing to change my orientation. Marla, however, is strongly heterosexual. The physical changes of a vagina instead of a penis, large breasts instead of a hairy chest, and smooth skin instead of five o'clock shadow has affected her at times. It is a testament to her love and commitment to our marriage that she and I are still together, having just celebrated our eleventh anniversary.

In conclusion, my life has drastically changed, yet improved. If I never transitioned I would not have had the platform to do some of the things that I've had an opportunity to accomplish. I would not be on the South Carolina HIV Prevention Council. I would not be a faculty member in the women's studies department. I would not be sought after to teach, lecture, and interview; and most importantly I would not be in a position to offer a positive and successful role model for other transgenders in the state and region. I never wanted to be a girl when I began this but I cannot imagine ever not being a girl now.

8

Nick and Mark

Nick Laird

Sometimes, just once in a while, when we're perched at each end of the sofa, pecking away at the dinner on our plates, watching the news on telly, I'll look over at Mark without him noticing. He'll have this content expression on his face and it's like I see all of him in those moments. I see him and can even picture him as a wee boy sitting in exactly the same position with his back straight and his knees together, chewing his food in the same neat, precise way he eats. I see him and feel how much he deserves to be loved, and I love him. In those moments I get such a warm, protective, feeling towards him that it actually brings tears to my eyes. It's beautiful.

On the other hand, sometimes he is a complete pain in the arse. For instance, he has to have the mugs in the cupboard placed in a particular order, which I have never been able to master and actually have no desire to master either. It suits me just fine to let him put the dishes in the cupboards the "right" way. His harder-to-love characteristics also include this annoying habit where he makes a sound that comes from the back of his throat and can only be described as a kind of internal alien-trying-to-break-out-of-body sort of noise. Not pleasant. The funny thing is that I have grown quite fond of Mark's annoying alien noise.

Mark is not perfect and from the tips of my toes to the top of my head I am delighted he is not perfect. I am delighted because I am well aware of my own imperfections. Had Mark been narrating this story he might have told you that I am forever putting things in the wrong cupboards, causing him to have to search high and low for some utensil he needs. He might have mentioned a few other imperfections I may have, which I will leave out of the story since it is me writing it. Obviously I will be giving myself the privilege of portraying myself in a, perhaps slightly biased, good light. I am not perfect and neither is Mark, but we do have—if not a perfect—a fantastic relationship. I love him and I know he loves me.

Before I met Mark, I had resigned myself to living a single life with a few friends for occasional company and masturbation for a sex life. My life lacked the intimacy I desired, but I had accepted that nobody would want to be with someone like me and, I would even go as far as to say I was generally quite happy. I had been taking testosterone injections for a year and was still getting such a kick out of my own developing male sex characteristics that it would have taken much more than a simple lack of intimacy in my life to bring me down. I had accepted being single and understood that there would be no one out there desiring a man like me—a man with a clitoris. Mark had no idea. He assumed I had a penis and I assumed he would only have a relationship with someone who had a penis. Not that I was consciously thinking about what Mark wanted, or what he thought.

When I was introduced to Mark by a mutual friend it did not occur to me in the slightest that we would ever be together. There was certainly no love at first sight going on. I was so switched off to the possibility that it never would have occurred to me to fancy him. I liked him immediately though and we became friends very quickly. I did not tell him about me being trans at first because, even though my close friends knew, I was enjoying meeting new people and just being accepted without having to justify my gender to people with a need to place me in a category. Since taking testosterone I found socializing a lot easier than I ever had before and my confidence was growing by the day. I always knew I would eventually tell Mark about my trans status if we remained friends. I feel that my trans experience is far too big a part of my life to not be out to friends about it. Generally, most people who know me know I am trans, but in the first couple of years of taking testosterone I was a lot more reticent about telling people.

About three weeks after I was introduced to Mark, he invited me and two other friends to his flat for a bite to eat. I know now that Mark fancied me and that was why he invited us, but at the time I was completely oblivious to this. I saw Mark as a very warm, kind, friendly man, which he is, but I was unaware at the time that he was trying to impress me. I was impressed as it happens. It turned out that Mark's bite to eat was one of the tastiest, best presented bites to eat I had ever had. He is a fantastic cook. His wee studio flat in the trendy West End of Glasgow in Scotland was all cosy with ambient candle light, a creatively homemade Christmas tree, soft music, and the smell of strong coffee. I sat on the sofa beside Mark and the conversation flowed between us. I felt comfortable. Later that night, when I was back at home in my own bed, I fantasized about Mark. It was, of course, just a fantasy. I knew Mark, a gay man, would never be interested in me. I thought he might possibly find me attractive with my clothes on, but definitely not if he knew what was under my clothes.

A few days later Mark phoned to tell me he had been given two tickets to see *Sing-a-Long to The Sound of Music* at the Theatre Royal and asked if I wanted to go with him. He had borrowed his neighbor's big swanky car with heated seats and would pick me up. Later I found out that this was Mark asking me out on a date with him. Since he did not explicitly mention that it was a date I had no idea. I read it as I saw it. He had free tickets and his neighbor was friendly. I assumed he asked me to go rather than anyone else because he saw me as someone who would enjoy a camp show. I did enjoy the show actually. Mark came back to my house afterwards for coffee (this is not a euphemism) and once again the conversation flowed, but nothing else happened. I liked him a lot, but since I knew he would not be interested in me, I was happy enough to have met such a nice new friend.

During the first few weeks of January I saw Mark most days. It was not always just the two of us, but we did start to meet on our own. The first time I realized my feelings for Mark was on a beautiful bright, crisp, cold Saturday afternoon. I met Mark in town for a coffee. We were having such a nice time talking to each other and after our coffee we walked the couple of miles from the City Centre, through Kelvingrove Park and back up to Byres Road in the West End. Later in the afternoon he asked me if I wanted to go back to his flat. I had to get home for my dog so I left Mark on Byres Road and took the underground home. It was when I was home, sitting in my room, just me and Floyd (the dog), I realized I was wishing Mark was with me. He was constantly on my mind and I was experiencing a very strange feeling, like part of me was missing when he was not with me. I phoned him and casually invited him over to my house if he had nothing else to do. He was over within the hour.

Even although we had only known each other for just over a month I felt like I had known Mark a lot longer. I wanted to tell him about my trans status because we had talked so much about our lives and I felt a huge part of my story was missing. For example, he knew that I had previously been in a relationship with a woman for seven years, but he did not know that relationship had been with the lesbian woman I was still living in the same house with. I wanted to be able to be open with him about my whole life. All I had to do was find the right time to tell him. Unbeknown to me, Mark also had something he wanted to tell me and it was his disclosure that opened the door for mine.

One evening when I met Mark I asked him how he was, as I would usually do, and usually he would say he was fine, but on this particular occasion he burst out crying. Not being much of a crier myself, I was surprised and worried that something dreadful had happened to him. We sat down on a nearby staircase and Mark told me he was crying happy tears because he had just received results from the hospital that day that the new combination of HIV drugs he was taking were working extremely well. I had previously wondered if Mark perhaps had HIV because he worked in the field and he had talked knowledgeably about HIV in general on a few occasions. What I could never have comprehended was that he had been living with HIV since the 1980s. His first partner died when Mark was only twenty-seven years old and then Mark had spent most of the 1990s expecting to get ill and die too. I had been too busy thinking about how complicated and difficult my own life had been to contemplate the possibility that Mark's life was also complicated and difficult. His disclosure meant our relationship had reached a new, deeper level of openness and trust and I knew I needed to tell him about me.

I decided not to use the words transsexual or transgender because they are often misinterpreted, or can be interpreted in different ways by different people. I once told an acquaintance that I was transsexual (I no longer use this term to describe myself) and he later made some reference to me as someone who "dressed up in women's clothes." At the time, I was baffled as to why he had thought such a thing, but I soon realized he had no idea any other trans identities exist and made assumptions based on his own limited knowledge. Incidentally, a man I know, when wearing a little black dress, was asked by a complete stranger, "Why are you wearing women's clothes?," his reply was "They're not women's clothes, they're mine."

Anyway, I did not want Mark to misunderstand what I was saying to him, so I told him I had been born with a female body. I could not think of a simpler way of putting it. I could see from Mark's expression that he was surprised and he told me he was. This was something that had never even crossed his mind. No matter how closely he looked, with my clothes on, there had been no signs for him to read. I had been taking testosterone long enough to be unnoticeable. Also, some of the signs I sometimes notice in some trans men are not very noticeable in me. For example, I am not particularly short for a man in western Scotland, I always had relatively narrow hips, biggish hands and feet and a kind of square jaw line. Even before testosterone I was often read as male anyway, so I was not surprised that Mark was surprised. I expected it.

He asked me what surgery I had had done and was even more surprised when I told him I had nothing done. I was skinny and had such a flat chest it was unnoticeable. Also, I wore a packer at that time, so I did look as though I had a cock. However, I was basically telling him I had tits and a vagina and I knew at this point that any interest he may have had in me would be gone. By telling each other these things about ourselves we had reached a deeper level in our friendship but, as far as I was concerned, we were never going to be more than just friends. It was not possible.

A week or so later, one evening when Mark had been round at my house watching a film, everything changed. He was about to leave to go home and was perched on the arm of the couch looking slightly nervous when he told me he really liked me and wanted to be with me. I was absolutely shocked, stunned, and surprised at this revelation. Mostly though, I was just terrified. I wanted to jump up and shout "YES," but I was scared and extremely cautious. I did say yes that night, but told him I needed the rest of the night to think about what he had said. We did not kiss or anything. I think we were both too nervous. I was relieved when he left and I am sure he was too.

I hardly slept that night. I lay thinking and, characteristically, worrying. I became convinced that Mark only thought he wanted to be with me because he had not seen me naked. The worst thing was that I was unsure if I would ever be able to test this theory because I felt so uncomfortable at the thought of him seeing me naked. I knew that Mark completely accepted me as a man the way things were and I did not want his view of me to change. That night I also had to admit to myself that I had some worries about Mark having HIV. I was not so worried about transmission because I was well aware of how HIV is transmitted and how to avoid transmission. I was more worried about starting a relationship with someone who could get ill or die. It did not take long for me to come to the conclusion that everyone dies, most often through being ill, and if I went through my life not getting close to anyone just in case I lost them at some point, I would not be living a life at all. He was healthy anyway. However, the following day I still told Mark that I thought it would be best if we remained just friends.

The next couple of weeks were slightly awkward between us. Mark backed off a bit, obviously trying to respect my wishes, but I was feeling like I had made a big mistake. I wanted him to still want me and to see me as a man even if we had sex together, but I was too insecure to let that happen. It is not that I am uncomfortable with my genitals these days, but I was then. I actually like my genitals now. I have come to an understanding that my genitals don't have a gender, they are just genitals, part of my body and, since I am a man, my genitals are part of a man's body. I understand how difficult it is for most people to get their heads around that idea, but it makes sense to me.

Ever since I was a small child I was always baffled by rules that seemed ridiculously nonsensical. The rule I found most ridiculous of all was that I had to have a penis to be a boy. Why? There is no logic to this rule for me. It is not that I am particularly rebellious when it comes to rules generally. I actually enjoy rules when they have a purpose that makes sense and are not about oppressing humanity. I did not credit Mark with the ability to be able to understand my viewpoint. It is not that I felt he would be less understanding than anyone else. It might have been a bit arrogant of me, but I never really expected anyone to understand. This was only because I had never found another human being who could see what was so clear to me. As far as everyone else was concerned there was something wrong with me for not conforming to the gender rules. As far as I am concerned there is something wrong with the rules in the first place. I even had to lie to doctors to get prescribed testosterone or, at least, I felt that I had to lie because I was scared they would not prescribe testosterone, which I desperately wanted to take. I pretended to want phalloplasty because I knew they could accept I was a man without a penis, but that they could not accept me as a man who did not want one. I felt I had to want one.

Anyway, the awkwardness between Mark and I was a bizarre mixture of neurosis and sexual tension. Mark had his neurosis too, but given the nature of neurosis, I was only focused on my own. I was unaware that Mark was feeling rejected and unattractive and thinking nobody would ever want him. If I had known, I would have told him that I found him incredibly sexy and that I was constantly thinking about him.

We nearly got together the night before we got together. It was a Saturday night and we were at a cheesy pop party. Mark was in the kitchen making what everyone there agreed was the best buffet ever. He wanted to do the food because he does not like dancing and does like making food. I love dancing, especially to cheesy pop songs, so I spent the evening on the dance floor. At the end of the evening I went to help Mark clean up, even although he had already done most of it because he is organized enough to cook and clean dishes at the same time. Most of the pots and pans belonged to Mark and I offered to help him carry them home, mostly because I did not want to go home to my own house without spending time with him that night. We were all set to go when a friend offered to drive Mark back to his flat with the pots and pans and was baffled as to why I still felt I had to help. Obviously there was no need for me to help Mark now that someone with a car could help him, but I knew he wanted me to go with him and I did.

That night, sitting close together on Mark's sofa, I felt it was inevitable that we would have sex. There was just something about the atmosphere. Maybe it was because I could hear my own heart beating, or the way Mark was looking at me, or the lighting and music, or maybe it was the porn magazine we were looking at together. The problem was that both of us were too scared to make the first move because each of us feared rejection for different reasons. Eventually, about four in the morning, I got a taxi home feeling unbelievably frustrated. We had not even kissed.

The next day, Sunday, February 11, 2001, we were both booked to go to some alternative therapy type course. The course turned out to be a bit scientifically questionable, but it was the perfect catalyst for initiating sex. I suppose that made it therapeutic after all. The course started early and I was running late due to going to bed so late and then not being able to sleep when I did go. I had to get a taxi. It was in that taxi that I acknowledged I was in love with Mark. The taxi passed him walking up the hill towards the flat where the course was being held, and I watched him out of the window and just knew that I was in love. I was excited to see him.

The course was all about crystals and energy. I went through a wee phase of being curiously, although sceptically, interested in this sort of thing because I was friends with an amazingly eccentric couple who had a kind of charismatic charm about them. Of course, they were also completely deluded and believed they could morph into aliens and all sorts of nonsense, but they were fun and harmless; although given other circumstances, Mikhail, as he called himself, could possibly have been a psychotic cult leader. I have no idea what happened to them. They just disappeared in a mysterious sort of way, although someone later told me they had moved to the seaside (very mysterious indeed).

Later that evening, Mark came back to my house under the auspice of practicing crystal healing on each other. We were in my bedroom with the relaxation music playing softly in the background and ambient candlelight. Mark was lying on his back on my bed letting me place crystals on his chakras. I started by placing a purple stone on his forehead, a blue one on his throat, green on his chest, yellow on his belly, orange on his abdomen and then I went to place the red and could see from the bulge in his jeans that his energies were already flowing quite nicely in that department. I unbuttoned him and put my hand in his pants.

It was all a bit of a fumbling, rushed, intense experience. I can remember looking down at Mark's face thinking he looked like he was enjoying himself and also thinking, "I can't believe I am actually fucking." I had been worried I would never have sex with another human being ever again and was feeling tremendously lucky to be doing it. It all ended rather abruptly though, due to the bed being old and squeaky, the walls in the house being paper thin, and Alison, my ex-girlfriend landlady banging on the door shouting "BE QUIET!" Just to clarify, Alison and I had been separated for some years and she had been through a good few relationships with other people since. It was not that I was being insensitive. I had heard her having sex through the thin walls too.

Mark had to leave very early the next morning because he had an early flight to catch to London for some freelance work he was doing there. He was away for ten days, which turned out to be a good thing because I felt those ten days gave me time to absorb what had happened. We talked on the phone and e-mailed every day. I was excited about him coming home and wanted to make it special. Mark had previously told me during one conversation that he loves when snowdrops start appearing because they keep him going through the rest of the winter knowing spring is on its way and that the daffodils will be out soon. The morning of the day Mark was due back, when walking the dog in the park, I dug up a few snowdrops with a tablespoon and put them into a tin I was using as a plant pot. I wanted the snowdrops to be a symbol of the optimism I had about our relationship. I took the snowdrops with me to Mark's flat. I had already agreed I would go to his flat before he got back to put the heating on and make the place nice and cosy. I sat waiting for him feeling excited, happy, and hardly able to believe my luck. We had an amazing time when he arrived home.

Everything was very intense for the first few months. I probably had more sex in those first few months than I had had during the rest of my entire life. It was fantastic. Being happy with Mark was probably what helped me to not be so upset with some of the negative reactions I was getting from some people about my relationship with Mark. My dad, who had a very hard time coming to terms with my transition, was confused by my relationship with Mark and made some pretty ignorant comments. He asked me why I would go to the bother of transitioning if I was going to end up being with a man anyway and said Mark was not really a gay man if he was with me. His views seemed to me to sum up how most of the world tends to think of sex and gender. I sometimes feel overwhelmed by how oppressive that feels. Our love felt bigger to me than the labels people wanted to limit us with.

Now, six years later, we have a strong, caring, close relationship and a comfortable home together. We get on remarkably well with each other and rarely argue. I think this is because we talk to each other. Our relationship began with open, honest communication, and I feel it has sustained us and helped us respect each other's feelings. We have had some amazing times together, like the week we spent living on a boat on the Canal di Midi in the South of France, but overall our lives are just wonderfully ordinary. We go to work, watch telly, go shopping and all the usual everyday stuff. I especially love a Saturday night when Mark cooks a delicious meal and then we sit playing scrabble and drinking cocktails until late.

9

Beyond Gender and Sexuality

Debra Hastings

My name is Debra, but everyone calls me Debs. At the time of this writing I am fifty years old. I live and work as a gay male but strongly identify as a straight female. I have always been feminine, never effeminate. I have always been open about who and what I am. I don't think I could hide it if I wanted to. And because my femininity comes naturally to me, other people pick up on that and react accordingly. Even when dressed in male attire, I am often mistaken for a woman. I find most people, including straight guys, subconsciously relate to me as a woman.

When puberty hit, I assumed I was gay as I was strongly attracted to men. As a youngster, I had crushes on male teachers, actors, and pop stars. During my teen years, I went through agony desiring other males but could never express or act on my desires. Because of the ignorance and homophobia of the time and place—early 1970s, small bush town in Australia—my sexuality was a deep, dark secret. In due course, I moved from the bush to Sydney where I learned about hormones and sex-change operations; transsexuals became my closest friends. I discovered that my sexual identity wasn't the same as my gender identity; that there was an almost limitless spectrum of how we labeled ourselves. Nevertheless, I hesitated to call myself a transsexual, chiefly because I didn't have the guts to do what my friends had done—abandon their male lives and live as women. I saw the hassle they went through every single day; they couldn't even go to the corner shop to buy a loaf of bread unless they looked perfect. The object of their lives was to look "real" and not get "sprung" as a man in drag. It was 1978 and no one in the everyday straight world knew what a transsexual was. Discovery of your biological gender would have met with derision and probably violence. That was not the sort of life I wanted to lead.

I lacked the confidence to take that step and live as a female although every fiber of my being told me that was what I was. I was tall, slim and lightly built with long, flowing blonde hair. I guess I was the perfect androgyne and I learned to accept that was how it would always be. And so I chose to live as what I called a "half-half," living and working as a male but dressing up every chance I got. It was a Dr. Jekyll and Miss Hyde lifestyle but it suited me and I was happy. Once I discovered the power of my female self, my sex life exploded. Dressed as a woman, I frequented straight venues and had sex with many an unsuspecting Aussie bloke, although I always divulged my true biology to any potential lover before sex took place. I wanted each guy to accept me as both the female they saw and were attracted to, as well as the boy's body that was revealed when my clothes came off. It was a strategy my trannie friends were horrified by, but it worked for me.

And so I happily lived my half-half life. Life was an adventure and I had a ball. I more or less partied nonstop, enjoying the best of both worlds—attracting straight and bi men when dressed up, or by taking advantage of my male body and enjoying the carnal delights of the gay scene. Romance was the only experience missing from my life but I had dismissed any dreams of a loving relationship as a lot of old rot, something not meant for me. Straight society conditions us to believe we are not complete unless we are in a relationship. It's all part of the human dualistic existence—black/white, male/female. Ugh, I quickly disassociated with that kind of thinking. I couldn't understand why some of my friends yearned to find Mr. Right. "Love 'em and leave 'em" was my motto. Life was a smorgasbord of men and sex. Why be tied to down to just one bloke? If, deep down, I harbored any notions of romantic bliss, I buried them beneath a facade of endless nightclubbing and sexual encounters.

I have always been a positive type of person, very rarely depressed or blue despite the underlying pain of not living to my full female potential. I simply accepted the life I had chosen for myself and got on with it. Moaning or slashing my wrists wouldn't change a thing. I am known to be a bit fiery, with a short temper and an acid mouth, but I am also a very loving and spiritual being. Like the rest of the human race, I'm a bunch of contradictions and the whole sexual/gender identity thing is all part of the mix.

In 1990 I moved from Sydney to London. New city, new life, but basically I adopted the same half-half lifestyle. I was convinced by then that I would never be in a loving one-on-one relationship with a man. And honestly, I never gave it another thought. I was quite content being single, thank you. I lived in the here and now and searching for a partner was not part of my life plan.

In London I discovered my love of all things fetish—the nightclubs, the clothes, the sex. It was all part of my personal evolution, but I seemed to be evolving in a different direction to most of the people around me. I had plenty of pals to go clubbing with but no one understood my passion for dungeons and domination, for boots and bondage. In an effort to cultivate friendships within the fetish scene and, to put it bluntly, get fucked in the process, I advertised in the personal ads section of a sex magazine. I presented myself as a male crossdresser seeking men or women for friendship, maybe more with the right person. There was no space in a small advert to discuss my gender identity so advertising as a transvestite was the easiest approach to take. I included a photo of myself looking as femininely sexual as possible in a black PVC corset and leggings and long black boots. I received many replies, but most were time-wasters. I had a few fun sexual encounters as a result of the ad but nothing to write home about.

One reply was from a lad called David. As he didn't enclose a photo with his reply, my flatmate advised me not to bother responding to him, not to take the risk that he was plug ugly. But I have good manners and as David had taken the time to write to me, I wrote back to him, telling him more about myself and inviting him to visit. When I opened the door to him I thought, "Oh, he's cute, thank God for that!" And he was very cute indeed with a sweet boyish face. He looked much younger than his thirty-one years. Naturally I was dressed up, not in fetish gear but a simple girly outfit. The first time he visited we didn't have any sexual contact, we just chatted. He said he was new to exploring his bisexuality and had only had a few encounters with transvestites, none of which, I gathered, were overly exciting. He was quiet and shy but easy to get on with. On his second visit we messed around and I was pleased to discover he was a very good kisser. He left, promising to call again soon. Two weeks later I hadn't heard from him, but I wasn't bothered. I figured he'd tried it and didn't like it. Besides, I had other ad replies to meet and play with.

But he did phone again and we saw more and more of each other. He explained that his silence after our first two meetings was because he was trying to deal with the feelings he had developed. He admitted he had been very attracted to me and wanted to be with me. So I took things slowly with him, being aware how new he was to all of this. We discovered the things we had in common besides the fetish sex scene. Soon we passed beyond being lovers to being friends and I introduced him to my circle of friends—gay boys, lesbians, trannies (pre and post op). At first I was worried he wouldn't fit in, given his timidity and lack of experience, but he turned out to be very personable and sociable in my friends' company. We went everywhere together; to movies, to gigs, to sci-fi conventions. It was both obvious and subtle, our coming together—obvious when I noticed in my diary how often I was seeing him and subtle in that my emotions were developing at their own pace. David may have been aware of the true nature his feelings, but I was ignorant of mine.

He was very affectionate, always holding my hand or cuddling me. As I wrote in my diary at the time "tenderness is just as lovely and just as needed as passion." We spent many an hour just curled up in bed, cuddling and kissing, dreamily content being with each other. I simply liked being with this boy. He was different than most men I had been with. He was well mannered and considerate. He didn't have any rough edges that most men possess, and he had a calmness about him that complimented my fast-paced spirit. He was so grounded while I was usually in a frenzy about one thing or another. We were opposites in many ways.

And being with him led to a surprising discovery about myself—I liked being dominated by him. Now ordinarily, no one tells me what to do, in or out of bed. The worst thing a man can do is put his hands on my head and push me down on him. No matter how gorgeous and sexy he is, that one act of dominance kills every ounce of passion in me. But not so with David. He is the one male I will let control me. It appeared we were both learning things about ourselves as we grew closer together.

The big test of our new "relationship" came when I allowed him to see me out of drag, sans make-up, as just another guy. But it made no difference to him. He treated me the same and felt the same about me. I was pleased.

Now I might add that all during this phase I was having sex with other guys, other ad replies. However, alarm bells started ringing when I found myself wishing I was with David rather than whichever guy I was bonking at the time. I didn't question those feelings any further, just pushed them out of my mind.

Six months after our first meeting he said those three little words to me—"I love you." I laughed and dismissed his words immediately. He's just a little straight boy fascinated by the whole trannie/fetish thing, I told myself. He had a crush on me, that's all, and would soon get over it. I steadfastly ignored the times when we were cuddled up together and "I love you" was on the tip of my own tongue, aching to be voiced. But I swallowed those words and pretended we were just friends who had sex.

Just as I was having sex with others, I urged David to explore his sexuality and meet other trannies/TVs/women, whatever turned him on. Then one day, not so long after he had declared his feelings for me, he told me he had "had some fun" with another transsexual and I felt as if I had been punched in the stomach. I was shocked, hurt, and in pain. That was what it took for me to realize I loved him, just as he loved me. I stopped fighting my inner feelings and gave in to the flood of emotions that inundated me. And so we became a couple.

It took a long time for me to settle into our relationship. David didn't have much difficulty adapting, he knew what he wanted and just went for it. I questioned everything. How could he, a cute straight guy eleven years my junior, love me, a forty-something bloke who liked to throw on a frock. I doubted my own gender identity and saw myself as an ugly old man in drag. I was scared that once I had given in to my feelings for David, he would tire of me and leave me. Neither of us believed in open relationships, so how could he commit to me when it would mean giving up sex with women? And would I, who had had a constant stream of casual lovers, be satisfied with just the one guy? Sometimes I thought my head would explode and I took it all out on poor David.

To make matters worse I decided to start taking hormones. I had always been curious as to what my life would have been like had I taken them in my twenties. Would I have been much more feminine? I knew one thing—I wanted to be as feminine as possible for David. I wanted to stun him with my girly image so that he never looked at the "real thing" again. Our fledgling relationship became very rocky because of my insecurity. I was paranoid and jealous, suspicious every time he so much as glanced at a woman. I argued and yelled and cried. After every tantrum David quietly reassured me that he really did love me and wanted to spend the rest of his life with me.

Eventually life settled down a bit, but it took a tempestuous twelve months to happen. I grew to accept that even an in-betweenie like myself could be loved. All the clichés about being in love suddenly made sense to me—they were no longer clichés but facts of life. We dated for three years, then bought a home together and haven't looked back. I believe that the fact that we didn't move in together straight away helped our relationship enormously. We had those three years to learn about each other, our habits, our likes and dislikes. He saw how I lived my mixed gender-bender lifestyle and I saw how he was coping with being with me. And when we weren't together, we had space to breathe and to process our development. We also missed each other greatly and could hardly wait to meet up again.

I have come to accept that David loves me whether I am en femme or lounging around the house in jeans and t-shirt. He has shown a level of commitment and devotion I would never have expected to inspire. I don't need a sex-change operation to keep him, nor do I need it for my own sanity. We have moved beyond sexual and gender identities, beyond the physical boundaries of our bodies. Ours is a relationship of the soul.

My friends readily accepted David as one of the gang and when we traveled to Australia my family welcomed him warmly. David has no family. His parents are deceased and he has lost contact with the few relatives he had. He is a very private person and to this day only a few of his friends know about me. His colleagues at work don't know I exist. That's fine by me. I respect his feelings on the subject.

As soon as UK law changed, allowing same-sex partners to form civil partnerships, David and I knew it was something we wanted to pursue. So we had our "wedding" on a sunny June day and are now in a legally recognized union with the same rights as heterosexual couples. Just think, I not only have a loving partner but am now officially "married" to him. We've both come a long way from that first day we met. I didn't think having our relationship formalized would make much difference to the way we feel about each other, but it did. It is hard to describe in words just how it has affected us; suffice it to say it has deepened our love and commitment to one another.

We have reached a plateau in our relationship; that is not to say it is stagnant or dull. We have both adapted to a life together with both of us making lifestyle changes. We have grown and evolved with each other and now share a domestic contentment that I never would have thought possible for someone like me. We have our ups and downs, but we very rarely argue. I believe ours is a fairly unique relationship. To the outside world I guess we appear as a gay male couple but as I said earlier, we ourselves have passed beyond those sorts of labels.

What does the future hold for us as a couple? Who knows? As long as we face it together, that's all we want.

10

From Russia With Love

Orsekov Dan

I first fell in love with a girl when I was five years old. She had beautiful black hair, brown eyes, and a nice smile. She also was my first disappointment after I stole away from our house to spend around thirty minutes with her. I even played with her stupid dolls just to stay close to her, but I encountered her indifference. "Oh, you," she said, standing with some boys. The disappointment quelled the need in me and I ceased to be interested anymore.

When I was ten I fell in love with a girl who was my distant relative. We only met in a village when on vacation visiting our grandmothers. I wrote her verses and climbed trees and picked apples for her. I nearly drowned trying to rescue her stocking that had fallen in the river. She spoke to me about discos and boys, but did not respond to my affection even though I told her stories about different books and astronomy. What was worse was that her girlfriends made fun of me, laughing about me talking about such things. It went on for five years and even the fact that she got married and gave birth to a child did not help me to give up the silly habit of looking at her adoringly and being jealous of her husband. She still does not know anything about my feelings, as I never disclosed them.

Then I met a girl named Jenya in high school. For the first time I understood what it is like to want someone and spend sleepless nights dreaming about a kiss or something more. By then I thought that I must be a lesbian and it seemed logical because I was a biological girl who loved girls. That realization did not surprise me. There was no shock or self-denigration. Everything was simple; after all, surely that would be my natural path, all things considered. Having been drinking with friends one night we walked home together discussing this and that and I went and admitted my love for her. It all came out quite naturally and one day while walking home from school I suggested that we kiss. She responded that she would rather be just friends but I cursed that day.

By the time I went to the university, my father's attitude towards me was going from bad to worse. After the collapse of the Soviet Union, his beliefs grew much stronger and he decided to become a devout and true Muslim. I did not share his beliefs, happy just to live my life following simple concepts such as not killing, stealing, or being unkind or evil towards other people.

My father told me every day, "You should be as a girl, put on female clothes, do not walk at night—you should be home at 7 p.m., grow your hair," and so on. He made it his business to tell me those things over and over again. Eventually I left home in my third year of university. My brother beat me up and I was left without money, clothes, or any means of support, leading to a very difficult, hard, and impoverished two years. Without money or my diploma, work was very hard to come by and I ended up being taken in by various friends, with no kind of security. I turned to alcohol and sometimes took drugs and seemed to find myself actively joining the lesbian community. For the first time I felt like a fish in water, but although I looked for a girlfriend, I just could not find the one.

I had a lot of sex at that time but no real emotional connections and perhaps I was not allowing myself to feel anything. Life was full of vodka and playing around but I really did not seem to learn anything and I remember I had a constant headache; maybe it was my unconscious telling me something. My father became ill and his hair went gray, all apparently because of me. There was hope that I might even marry a gay man and live with him separately so the family could be happy that I would appear normal. I never took the bait and avoided going along that road because I knew in my heart of hearts it was really an impossible solution.

At the time I was very afraid that my brother was searching for me and I had nightmares that he would find me, beat me up, and strangle me so I would not be an embarrassment to the family anymore. I am not a coward but I had no wish to be maimed, crippled, or humiliated more than I had been already. I know my mother suffered badly because of me but I was unable to offer her comfort. Of course a woman should raise her children according to Muslim customs, and if there is something wrong with them, she is as guilty as much as they are. My younger brother and sister knew nothing of "how ugly and wrong" I was.

Then there was the depression I suffered, and I cannot explain what the reason was for it but I was at times deeply depressed. A few times I moved back home and my father and I decided to begin everything again. He selected other tactics to influence me and even though they were not physical, they were painful through emotional blackmail. It was all about morality and the rights or wrongs of me, though more about the wrongness of me.

I tried to commit suicide because of the constant mental pressure I felt I suffered and a parting with the girl with whom I had begun a serious relationship. That was a long year full of depression and useless sufferings, half in and half out of the ideas of whether to live or die and ultimately I ended up in a psychiatric clinic. My father was one hundred percent sure I was crazy but he ceased to pressure me when I ended up in the clinic. However, my elder brother reacted differently, determined to reeducate me. He decided to destroy me both emotionally and physically, proving that I was an unnecessary dirty stain on our family's name.

My private life was promiscuous. One night I was with one girl, considering her the best, then she would annoy me. Then I would find another one and while she was my official girlfriend I would meet another one at a party and so on. By the time I was twenty-two years old I was tired and completely without hope of any kind of romantic relations. Then I spent a year where I just worked, devoting extra time to friendship and creativity. A whole year passed in chastity in an atmosphere of a monk's life with being really quiet and nothing disturbing me.

After a while I met a young girl to whom I first admitted that I am a guy "with some problems." I felt it was necessary to tell her that, because by that time I had heard of transgender and transsexual people. When I heard about these people I understood immediately what my problem was and my depression just vanished. Finally, I understood my predicament and my total unwillingness to connect with my own body.

Even though the relationship with that girl ended, it did not bother me that much because I was free from confusion and I was almost happy at the relief of at last being able to understand myself. It was almost like a lightbulb going on as I eventually started to understand how I needed to build romantic relationships for me. Since that time many things have changed in my mind. I finally understood that my life is my life and my parents have already lived their lives how they wanted. Now it was my turn and I could make my own choices about my own life.

It was tricky at times explaining to all my friends, including the gay and lesbian ones, who I really was. Gay people like people of the same sex and they like their own bodies, so I often faced such questions like "Why are you going to make such a drastic change?" Many found it funny, confusing, or simply insane. Many tried to make their views clear to me and I would laugh or get angry. It appeared much more difficult to explain it to the gays and lesbians than it did to the heterosexuals or bisexuals. When I started to communicate closer with other transgendered men, life became much easier for me as I did not have to go into huge explanations because they understood exactly what I was talking about and offered help but not judgment.

The situation with the family improved as they got used to my lifestyle, even asking sometimes, "When will you marry?" Mother, by the way, has understood to some extent. Somehow she understands that I am going to have an operation to change my sex. Her reasons for being more accepting are all reduced to the logic that it will be Allah who will punish me. Her belief is that we have been given life in one body and I should not change it, otherwise I will be in hell. For me they are all empty phrases. I did not kill anyone, steal anything, or hurt anyone. Why should I go to hell just because of the desire to be happy? Do not make me laugh!

Then I met Regina. She is younger than me. We met at a dinner party where there were four of us who were just hanging out, eating salad, and drinking beer. The dinner was given by a lesbian acquaintance who had invited two younger girls to join us. I was annoyed at first because I would rather have spent the time with her talking face to face about common friends. However, she had invited these two younger heterosexual girls who I initially found irritating. We were getting drunk and I did not say much but then one girl suddenly started smiling at me and I could not even remember her name.

Her smile was so sunny and friendly that it blinded me. I said to her, "I think I like you. You seem nice." She replied, "Really?" and smiled at me again. I was frankly surprised because in fact she was just some younger heterosexual girl. I had spent a year wearing the slogan "No sex or heart moves." I had not even had a date for three months and certainly was not ready to court someone and explain who and what I was. I was almost sort of hoping that she would not want to have a relationship with me.

Later in the evening we went outside to smoke a cigarette and I was just happy enjoying the intimacy, then she told me, "I saw you in my dream." I was shocked. It was almost like from that moment we were tied together with an invisible cord. When we went to bed together it felt so natural as if we had lived together for ten years. We decided that we should be together on my birthday and then she moved into my flat several days later. As we became closer, I understood in that moment that it did not matter how many girls I had been with before. Nor did it matter how many times I had tried to have really serious relationships with other women and failed. From the start, living together with Regina was a completely different thing. I could not even call her a girlfriend as it felt like she was my wife and so it was very different from anything I had experienced before.

From the first time she touched me, I shuddered all over. It was unusual that someone could reach me in that way, instantly bypassing all my barriers. I would always report to her where I was going, with whom, and we went to all the parties together as a couple. That was strange and unusual for me and as a much of a surprise to me as to my friends, but I always wanted someone to be the other half of a relationship and it showed me a whole other side of life.

It was so clear from the start that she was ideal for me. She grew to easily understand and support me. I did not want to lose her but I knew I would be unable to change the way I was. Eventually she decided to accept me as I am. Selfish or not, I could only be me. We had some quarrels around it in the beginning but then they passed.

There was something else. We had a period when our characters collided. It usually involved alcohol and after drinking we were both the worse for it. I carped on at her and she reiterated with equal fury. Once she got so upset that she fainted. Or we swore at each other and she would run out of the flat into the street in the middle of the night and I would run after her. I was initially irritated with many features of her character, thinking her silly and aspiring to be an "ideal person." I could not understand that she has her own originality and individuality. Later she told me that she understood all our quarrels were certainly because of inexperience, youth, pride, and whims.

At that time I lived in a one-room apartment with two girls whom I had known for a long time, so we were great friends. I always had clean clothes and supper ready (just as at mother's home) when Regina moved in. I was reticent initially about losing my freedom. I guess it is a certain sort of shock for those of us who are used to living alone and used to relating to others as a single person.

I never spoke with her about love because I had given up on the idea of being in love with another person. I wanted the type of marriage built on respect and common sense. I was undoubtedly thrilled that as we progressed, she became a girl who had no doubt of me as a boy. She grew to fully understand my "problems" with my body and that I would be seeking to physically correct them in years to come. I do not think it could be easy for a woman to live with the man who has constant problems with jobs and who constantly experiences rudeness and embarrassment in society.

Regina is Asian so she knows Muslim holidays and customs. We grew up in similar families that are typically standard Muslim families of Kyrgyzstan. Our families know little about us at the present time. The only other relative who knows that I am female to male (FTM) is my aunt, so I can visit her and be myself. She also knows that Regina is my partner and has no problem with our relationship. I have introduced Regina to my mother, younger brother, and sister. They consider that we are close friends, but I do not doubt that my mother guesses the nature of our true relationship. I have met some members of Regina's family and because of the way I am presenting, they think I am her boyfriend. Her mother thinks I am a teenager who is much younger than her daughter by many years.

We have lived together for two years now. I work on the computer in a little shop. It is hard for me to find a job as I face negative attitudes toward my identity. Unfortunately, employers look at my passport and ask stupid questions. We worked together in the grocery shop in autumn 2006. That was my first job where I was officially Daniyar (my Kyrgyz name). Regina helped me by giving me confidence not to be afraid of telling who I am.

Sometimes people in confusion call me "she." I used to keep silent but now I explain to them how they are wrong. I cannot buy beer in some markets because I look so young so I have to ask Regina to buy it for me and that really get gets on my nerves. Many men show aggression towards me, thinking I am a pushy teenager. It is upsetting at times because I often do not get the respect of being my real age but at least they are taking me to be a boy.

Since Regina and I started to live together we have lived in four different apartments. Now we live in a three-room apartment with three other people. Regina and I have got ourselves a cat who we learned to be parents to. We sit playing with her till late at night just talking and discussing all the things in life that interest us. In the morning we tell each other our dreams, trying to analyze them, and to understand what we worry about. I write stories, Regina writes verses. We show each other our new stories and poems. We plan to one day publish a book of our creations and we definitely would like to travel together in the future.

Regina is studying to be a lawyer at the university. She is eager to receive her diploma quickly and to fight to protect the rights of GLBT groups. In her spare time she does sensitivity trainings at schools and universities to familiarize people with GLBT issues. Sometimes I write articles about transsexuals and I am going to distribute brochures on this theme to the centers that are engaged in running various helplines. I hope it will be helpful to some young transgender people who call helplines looking for support, and psychologists could advise them that they are not alone, whether they are FTM or male to female (MTF).

When I go to the hospital I am frequently faced with misunderstanding and curiosity, the latter irritating me the most. There are eternal questions about what I am and why I am doing what I am, which upsets me but I am learning to ignore it. Life, I am hoping, is teaching me patience. If you know you are transgender then there can be many problems to face. Many of us get used to our families turning away and even some friends too. Sometimes I feel it a constant struggle. If you have no partner, who will be near to you even as your best friend? It can be hard.

Regina and I have divided family roles—with me working, and her taking care of the home as well as studying. She is happy engaged in domestic affairs such as cooking and cleaning. We frequently take long walks, meet friends, and simply spend pleasant times together as a couple. Now I am taking hormones and waiting for a diagnosis, I am so very glad to have a friend, lover, helper, wife, and relative all in one person.

11

Queerly Beloved: How a Lesbian Love Survived Transition

Jacob Anderson-Minshall

The standard arch of trans relationships—as portrayed in documentary films, biographical memoirs, and television specials—shows the heroine struggling to deal with the imminent and life-altering transformation of her partner (who insists on doing this to her despite the pain it causes). The couple announces their determination to stay together. Love will find a way. Fade to black. Cut to a year or so after transition and focus in on the trans person alone in the frame, their partner long gone.

It's been two years since I began my own transition and my partner of seventeen years is still by my side. When we set out on this path we didn't know there were others like us, but we've found that we are not alone. Like a growing number of other trans couples, we're breaking the rules, especially those that position the nontrans female partner as a powerless victim. We are forging our own path and demanding to be recognized as the queer couple that we remain, refusing to succumb to normative pressures that insist if we are no longer a lesbian couple, we must, by default, be a straight one.

I first met Diane at Idaho's first Gay Pride parade. She was a friend of a friend who I barely noticed—outside of her cut-up ACT-UP t-shirt that barely contained her large breasts and seemed a little more openly political than most Idahoan gays were willing to be. I was wearing a Lesbian Avengers t-shirt.

I met her again that weekend at a Queer Nation meeting she hosted and although I was with a hook-up and Diane appeared happily married to another woman, there was this undeniable connection between us. Every time our eyes met, it felt like lightning followed her gaze and disrupted the beating of my heart. She'd discarded the butchy t-shirt for tight-fitting clothes that hugged every curve of her voluptuous body.

I dismissed my interest. I didn't see how anything could happen between us. She lived in Boise, Idaho with a little queer family, while I lived four hours away in Pocatello. I went back to my life in Pocatello, attending graduate school classes and wallowing in a deepening unexplainable depression. I finally went to the school medical center and admitted my emotional state and ended up on a Prozac-like anti-depressant.

I didn't take well to the drug. I grew irritable and every muscle in my body seemed to tie itself into knots. I couldn't sit still. I started fantasizing about suicide. I grew increasingly erratic. Unable to tolerate sitting still for an entire fifty-minute class, I'd dart out in the middle of sessions. I'd just get up and leave all my books on the desk, my backpack nearby, and I'd go outside, cover my ears, and scream. Mostly no one seemed to notice. I begged the doctor to take me off the drug. He insisted that we just hadn't found an appropriate dosage and warned me if I stopped cold turkey, things could get worse.

One night I watched *Thelma and Louise* at the campus theater. The next day I impulsively decided to follow suit and drive my Ford LTD off a bridge. Each bridge I passed seemed to have some problem. Either the water was too low or the railing was too high. I kept driving, and in doing so, began to feel a relief at my escape. I ended up in Boise again, at Diane's home. She convinced me to flush the remaining supply of my drugs.

Despite the presence of her girlfriend, Diane (who I later discovered was in an open relationship) seemed intent on ratcheting up the sexual tension between us. I spent the night on their floor. The next day we went to see *Paris is Burning*. In the darkness of the theater Diane ran her hand up my thigh. She said she was going to visit me for a hook-up. As I'm rather obtuse, I assumed she was just toying with me. But she came to visit over Halloween weekend.

Although it was supposed to be a purely sexual thing I was hooked by the next morning. Still, she probably would have kept it a physical relationship if we hadn't fallen so hard for each other. Diane's the kind of modern sexually liberated girl who likes to leave her sexual conquests as soon as the act is over. She never spent the night with a one-night stand. Until me.

Since we lived six hours away from each other, getting together took an investment of time and energy and when she came to visit she stayed for the weekend. Today, she says, it was the intensive time we spent together that led her to fall so fast. For me it was all over the next morning. There was something about her still face in the morning light. I was compelled to trace every detail of her gorgeous lips, strong nose, and full eyebrows. And I was hooked.

COMING TOGETHER

A few short months later we moved to New Orleans with Diane's ex and her gay friend Jeff. Jobs were difficult to come by in the economically depressed south. After struggling with temp office jobs, we were all hired by a house renovation service to paint houses. We didn't get paid until the job was completed and sometimes that took a month or more. The heat of the summer was unbearable with 90 percent humidity. Unable to pay our electric bill, our power was shut off and we had no fans or air conditioning to cut the heat. The houses we worked on were air-conditioned and gave us our only relief from the sweltering summer.

As summer work died down, we fled New Orleans, returning to Idaho long enough for me to finish my graduate class work, then we tried the Big Easy again, before following Diane's job offer to the San Francisco Bay Area where we've lived for all but one of the ensuing years (when we once again tried our hand at Idaho).

During our first month in San Francisco, Diane and I lived out of our VW van with our Border Collie, Free. In the evening we drove to Half Moon Bay and stayed at a state park; during the day we parked down the hill from our jobs at Blush Entertainment (home of the lesbian erotic magazine *On Our Backs* and Fatale Video). Every few hours we'd dart out to move the vehicle and check on Free. Later we shared a tiny one-bed trailer, with Jeff, Free, and three cats. An hour outside of San Francisco, on the edge of a horse corral, deer ticks siphoned our blood, mice inhabited our silverware drawers, and flushing the archaic sewage system required manually lifting the effluent drainage hose to, uh, move things along.

Next we moved to a remote cabin in Pescadero where the water came out brown, the wood stove spewed black creosote, our landlord took up living in the crawl space, and during a storm a downed power line trapped us in the place for a week and a half. As cabin fever set in we begged Jeff and Reg, who were living in the Castro, to come pick us up and we hiked out to meet them. Diane, Free, and I crammed in the backseat of Reg's Geo Metro for the long ride into San Francisco. Rain came down in buckets. As we neared the city, a freeway sign describing the upcoming exits was blown off an overpass and landed on the road two cars in front of us. I was certain we were about to crash. Our friend Reggie deftly avoided the stopped vehicles in front of us by veering left and narrowly avoided slamming into the cement barricade. As we came to a rest I exhaled in relief. Then a pick-up truck rammed into us going 60 mph, totaled the Geo, and changed our lives.

That accident was to become the root of my ongoing chronic and disabling back pain, although it did not appear until later in what I like to call "the year of car crashes"—after we were rear-ended twice more within twelve months. Internal disc disruption made sitting and bending unbearable and soon landed me on disability. It took eighteen months for me to recover, during which time Diane was forced to support us on her meager lesbian publishing salary.

Nearly a decade later, after I'd had a new career as a park ranger, a work accident re-injured my back and sparked the chronic myofascial pain that—nearly four years later—still prohibits me from sitting, standing in lines, and participating in many "normal" life activities. Although I was covered under worker's compensation, long-term disability, social security, and state disability, the benefits have long since dried up and we are again surviving on Diane's salary. Living in the San Francisco Bay Area on one person's salary is an accomplishment. All the more so when that salary hails from an independent lesbian publication.

MAKING IT WORK

Love can't solve every problem and there have been times that we've taken our angst out on each other. But aligned together, we've overcome the difficulties life has thrown our way. Our bond has also enabled us to overcome our numerous differences. Diane is of mixed race, born in Los Angeles to working-class parents, but raised outside

Boise, Idaho by her white upper-middle-class grandmother and aunt. Meanwhile I'm a descendant of Germans, Brits, and Normans and my parents are middle-class academics. I grew up on a remote Idaho farm five miles from a town of 800. She's a tough, sexually adventurous, outgoing lesbian who likes being a girlie girl, while I'm sexually introverted; a soft butch turned nerdy man. We are both attracted to difference, and willing to work through some of our inherited baggage—and mock the rest.

I've become a relationship convert; a true believer; a prophesizer. I wasn't always this way. In fact, I was quite the opposite. Before I met Diane, my longest relationship had been a year (long distance) and I was not faithful. The rest of my two-dozen relationships fizzled out long before the three-month mark. It wasn't them, it was me.

Okay, some of it *was* them, but when you're too drunk, or needy, or whatever to notice that the woman you've just slept with is capital "C" crazy, and instead form some kind of compulsory relationship with her because you want to feel like the kind of gentleman who isn't just trying to get his rocks off but actually respects women, then you kind of have to take some responsibility for problems that arise.

Especially when it doesn't happen just once. When it's not just the girl who had a split personality, but also the girl who once got so upset about her ex-partner seeing someone new that she took a knife and slit her own belly from side to side. After a few of these hook-ups one has to realize that either a) all lesbians are crazy, or b) I attract very damaged individuals. I decided it was the latter. Plus, there were other parts of my relationship endings that were *all* my fault. I pushed women away. I didn't like them getting close and I'd start being an asshole so they'd dump me and I wouldn't have to be the bad guy.

So after all that, how did I know that Diane was the one? Hell, by the time I met her I didn't even believe in *the one* anymore. It's true that I fell for her hard and fast after we first started our affair. Still, it wasn't as though I thought then that we'd be together seventeen years and counting.

When the three-month anniversary came about, I felt my old issues coming up and we seemed to be having the same problems I'd had in the past. There were just two differences: (1) Diane wouldn't fall for any of my bullshit, and (2) in Diane I finally found someone who I wanted to work through my emotional baggage with. Like that now clichéd phrase, she made me want to be a better man. It was true. Every time I wanted to walk away—and I still had those feelings in the first year—this time I'd turn around, apologize, and make an effort.

It wasn't always easy. Since JoAnn Loulan's *Butch Femme Dance,* there has been an awareness of a well-documented pattern in lesbian couples. Dykes, she found, tended to break up at regular intervals, which she came to see as stressor points. Three months, six months, nine months, one year, three years, seven years, and so on.

There were struggles and difficulties in our relationship I didn't foresee. But what I discovered after sticking through the three, six, and nine-month periods was that the problems might have been cyclical but they were also temporary. If you hung around and worked on it long enough, it got better. In fact, it was only after these periods that I discovered new depths in the relationship.

Good relationships are like some kind of reverse atomic arithmetic where the total is less than the sum of the partners. We are two individuals and yet together we've become one coupled being. Sometimes Diane and I act as one. We share a history. Diane starts to tell a story about her childhood and then pauses, embarrassed when she suddenly remembers that it is my childhood experience she is remembering.

Many trans people have stories about not knowing anything about people transitioning, and the instant they did, they knew it was right for them. That wasn't the case with me. When I first came out as lesbian at eighteen, my mother asked, "Are you sure you just don't want to be a man?" While that was a rather abstract reference to transsexuals, during the mid 1990s there was a mini explosion of trans awareness in San Francisco and for a while you couldn't turn on a daytime talk show without seeing a trans pioneer like Stafford.

During that time period, Diane and I were busy starting and running *Girlfriends* magazine. I felt validated in my butch presentation. On my arm I had a sexy, totally stacked DDD, long-haired, red-nailed femme that any straight guy would desire. I wore men's clothes and occasionally packed. I thought this is what it meant to be a butch, just as I thought Diane's tomboy childhood, assertiveness, and success-driven nature was what it meant to be femme. Even when our *Girlfriends* co-founder, Heather Findlay, announced that her partner Sue was going to become a man, I didn't recognize myself within Sue's experience.

If it weren't for Diane, who knows if I'd ever have figured it out. Our relationship did provide me with deep happiness and a sense of wellbeing that probably served to postpone the gender issues that bubbled below the surface. It was when Diane was working on her anthology *Becoming: Young Ideas on Gender, Identity, and Sexuality* that I first began to identify with trans people. I began saying that if I'd been born a generation later, I'd probably be one of those genderqueer trans bois. I felt like it was a past opportunity, an option only for the young and I would have to wait for another lifetime to be a man. Six months later *Bitch* magazine asked me to review a number of new trans memoirs. During the writing of that piece, it all crystallized for me and I came out to myself and then to Diane. She already knew it was coming.

By the time the review went to print, I was no longer Susannah. Almost overnight I'd become Jacob.

BECOMING A MAN

Diane likes to say "when we transitioned" and people wonder why she says "we." She does so because she strongly believes that couples transition together and become in essence a *trans couple*.

When I first acknowledged my trans gender and my interest in transitioning, I was terrified about how Diane would respond and whether she would leave me. For her, that was never a question. Once I verbalized my feelings and desires, she immediately supported my decision and set about getting me through the transition. She bought me my new male wardrobe, grooming supplies, and even a pack and pisser.

Diane is an action-oriented woman. She doesn't want to sit around processing a problem, she wants to fix it. Once I verbalized my desire to transition, she set about making it happen. I was in therapy one week and having surgery soon after. I'm not saying she took me anywhere I didn't want to go, but I was frightened and tentative and would have stretched the transition out over years if she'd asked me to. But she didn't. If I was going to become a man, then she wanted to close the door on Susannah, as soon as possible.

That's not to say it wasn't a struggle for her or that she didn't mourn the loss of her wife. She did. She probably still does. But fortunately for me she didn't feel betrayed as my many of my female relatives who angrily denounced my decision to transition, demanding, "How could you do this to Diane?" For what it's worth, Diane is a strong and intelligent career woman and not the kind of woman who would go through life letting bad things be *done to* her by her life partner.

My decision to transition has already impacted Diane professionally. First, there was an employee (now no longer working with her) who made it quite clear that she would not work with me as a contributor. She also frequently hinted that a woman married to a man—albeit a trans man—was no longer a lesbian and should not be running the nation's largest lesbian magazine.

I'm happy to say that those vocally and subversively undermining Diane's role there are no longer with the magazine at her company. In addition, Diane's boss—a true friend—has been incredibly supportive of her, our relationship, and me personally.

I feel an allegiance and commitment to the lesbian community I came out in twenty years ago, but I recognize that as my transition progressed and I now pass more easily as male, I am less often recognized as an ally. Sometimes I'm a suspicious intruder. As Diane's partner, I go along with her to lesbian events. Lesbians seem to respond to me one of two ways, either they assume I'm a very butch lesbian (asking me things like, "Is that your *real* voice") or they eye me suspiciously, not quite sure what I'm doing there. When we were at a lesbian-owned B&B, Diane introduced me as her husband but apparently the owner couldn't process the lesbian married to a man thing and kept referring to us as "girls" even while calling me Jake.

Partly in response to the way "husband" throws people off and partly because husband doesn't seem to illustrate the realities of our relationship I asked that Diane start calling me her "partner." She's resisted. She called me "wife" for fifteen years. To now use "partner" seems like backsliding. She's trying it out, but she's not happy about it. It's possible that I worry about my trans gender impacting her career more than she does.

A QUEER MARRIAGE

When our relationship was described in the *New York Times* article "The Trouble When Jane Becomes Jack," readers and entertainment producers alike contacted us. They all wanted to know one thing—

how could Diane still insist on being called a lesbian when she was now with a man? But there is no reason for her to change her identity or orientation simply because I've decided to change [or reiterate] mine.

I explain it this way—if a straight woman sleeps with another woman it doesn't make her a lesbian. Despite her jocular insistence that she'll marry for money next time, in reality if Diane were not with me, she would be with another woman, not a man. But we've seen the way lesbians can ostracize a lesbian when she hooks up with a man. If they don't also ostracize us, would it mean that they disregard my masculinity, thinking that I'm not *really* a man?

Even as the femme in a butch-femme couple, Diane was often assumed to be a straight woman. When we took each other's names, we were most likely to be asked if we were sisters, despite looking nothing alike. We'd have to come out as lesbians repeatedly, frequently.

Now I'm taken as male and that *is* refreshing; it feels right, it feels like home. Still, we are more than a heterosexual couple but our queerness isn't visible. Diane doesn't always want to say, "This is my husband/partner Jake, he's a trans man," but without awkward statements like that how can we get others to understand the complexity of our relationship or identities?

Because I'm married to a woman, people assume I'm straight. Even trans men make this assumption. I take issue with that assumption for several reasons. First of all, I personally believe that when a female-born person is now a man, any sex with that person is queer. Second, a femme lesbian is not a straight woman and therefore sex with a femme lesbian is not straight sex. And third, I'm not straight— I'm *married*. Within the context of that monogamous marriage it doesn't matter that I find gay men hot or that I like watching gay porn or even that, never having had sex with a man, I'm intrigued and have fantasized about what it would be like (not every position, mind you). As a married, monogamous man, I take whatever erotic input I receive and express that in bed with my wife.

In a country where fifty percent of all marriages end in divorce, it goes without saying that relationships are difficult. Queer relationships are more so. There are innumerable systems in place to support heterosexual couplings, especially marriages. There are tax breaks, wedding registries, and divorce. Yes, even divorce. Because the intricacies of divorce law and the heart-wrenching and monetarily devastating divorce proceedings make separating difficult, this provides an impetus for heterosexuals to stay together.

For years gays and lesbians have been saying that civil unions are not equivalent to heterosexual marriage. Having had both, I can say that is true, but I don't know that legalizing gay marriage will resolve all the inequalities. Certainly, some people, like my parents who value the institution of marriage itself, will respect gays for having gone through the ceremony/commitment. It didn't seem to matter that we had been together sixteen years and been through multiple ceremonies including the Valentine's Day same-sex marriages at San Francisco's City Hall. Things changed with our legal marriage. My parents came to the wedding. They began to treat us differently.

But most of the differences came in the way strangers treated Diane and I both pre- and post-marriage. Store clerks "oooh-ed" and "ahhhed" about the upcoming nuptials. All it took was my male name and the simple word "husband" to persuade representatives of everything from credit card companies to HMOs to reveal personal information about my wife, which had previously been denied me as her registered domestic partner of fifteen years. In small, barely perceptible instances throughout the day our relationship is honored and respected now that we are "legally" married. But I imagine that many of those people who are supportive of us post-marriage would not be so friendly if the partners in question appeared to be of the same sex.

COMING OUT, STAYING IN

This fall we moved into a new apartment building. It was the first place we'd moved to since my gender/name change. We filled out the rental application with my masculine name and gender and submitted it, wondering if the trans issue would come up in the credit check. Although we'd always pointedly outed ourselves when we were at this stage as a lesbian couple, this time we decided not to mention it unless it did come up. When we came back to the apartment to fill out the rental agreement our landlord, a first generation Mexican American who still pronounces my name as Jack, said, "I don't know if anyone has ever told you this, Jack, but. . ."

Diane and I shared knowing glances, expecting this statement to end with "Your references insisted your name was Susannah," or "You look kind of like a girl." Instead, she said, "You look like Leonardo DiCaprio from *Titanic*." A smile crossed Diane's face. Her eyes told me she was amused, relieved, and happy. Diane is happy when people accept me as the man she sees me as. Although we're both proud of my trans identity, Diane knows that when people learn that I am female to male (FTM), they often respond as though I am not quite male after all.

Recently a lesbian filmmaker ignored me while she spoke with Diane who sat next to me at a banquet table. Diane introduced me as her partner, Jake, and mentioned that I was trans.

"You mean you used to be a man?" the woman asked.

"No, the other way around."

"You used to be a *woman*?" The woman was incredulous. She looked me over then added, "That is *so* hot." She tells us about finding Katastrophe, a hip-hop producer and trans man, attractive and questioning her sexuality—until she discovered he used to be female. Diane and I wince at the woman's assumption that trans men aren't really men.

Although during the first six months of my transition she eagerly told everyone from grocery clerks to phone servicemen that I used to be a woman, today Diane is happy when I'm accepted as a man, or a trans man, but not *less* than a man. She has no reservations when I'm taken as male. But sometimes I do. Not because I don't want to pass. In a perfect world, all trans people would pass as whatever gender they identified with, but they would never *have* to. If only we could be accepted as fully gendered and fully safe without passing, then we wouldn't feel pressured to do so. So, I do want to pass—at least in some situations.

Or maybe I don't. Isn't the idea of passing one that reflects someone's portrayal of something they are not being accepted as that thing? I am *not* not-a-man. I am a man. I want men to treat me as one of their own. I want to be accepted as male. But, sometimes when I am accepted as male, particularly when I'm in the company of Diane, I feel something else — shame perhaps. Because I know that my being seen, my becoming visible as a man comes at the price of *her* lesbian visibility. In the situations where I'm not out about my gender and my past, I drag her into the closet.

As a femme, Diane has frequently been mistaken for a straight woman. When I was a woman and we were together it helped reiterate her lesbian identity. But not now, when I'm with her, my gender is accepted. It's difficult enough that those who know of my transition use it to question her sexuality, but now my very appearance invalidates her sexual orientation.

I struggle to understand why femme is not widely recognized as the uniquely lesbian interpretation of a feminine gender expression that it seems so clearly to be. Certainly the heterosexual world doesn't seem to have a place for women who simultaneously command a sensual sexuality, feminist precepts, feminine attire, and an assertive nature.

Love may not conquer everything, but neither does transition destroy every relationship and leave the victimized female partner bereft. Rather than being the victim of my transition, Diane has taken an active role in orchestrating both my physical metamorphosis and the transformation of our relationship. Nor was she deterred by the struggles inherent in transformation or by the painful invalidation she's undergoing within some lesbian contexts. We may be legally married and together we may appear as a normative heterosexual couple, but we are far from straight.

12

Sex and the Single Trannie

Monica F. Helms

"NO! I refuse to believe you!"

"Sorry, Monica. Once you start hormones, you'll lose your libido."

"I will NOT let that happen."

"You'll have no choice."

"We'll see about that."

One may ask, "What does libido have to do with love?" This is, after all, an anthology of trans people and love, and very little about sexual desires. That may be so, but I cannot separate the strong connections between all of those parts of my personality.

Most people understand that humans are extremely complex biological organisms that have the capacity to experience a large range of emotions, including the elusive one known as "love." They also can feel a multitude of physical sensations and understand what they all mean, especially sexual pleasures. Over the course of the past decade, I've experienced love and sexual pleasures on so many levels that it would be hard to isolate one special moment or one special person. Others in this book may have a partner or someone special, but I don't. Yet, I have loved and lost enough times to know what the experience feels like.

While writing my autobiography in 2005, I had a chance to scrutinize the experiences I had with women while living as a man. I didn't have many encounters with women, so the ones I did have stood out rather vividly. A connecting thread between all of those loves began to emerge, surprising the hell out of me when it became obvious. This thread occurred because Mother Nature had endowed me with such a miniscule "tool" that it forced me to find more creative ways to satisfy women. Not surprising, many of those ways have been used by lesbians since the dawn of time. It appears that Mother Nature actually gave me a gift, preparing me for my future life as a lesbian.

As a man, I truly enjoyed making love with women and I enjoyed the pleasure they gave me. But, as I approached the time to start hormones, I became more and more worried that I wouldn't even feel like making love to anyone because of losing my libido. To not find intimacy exciting any longer sent a chill through the Italian blood coursing through my veins. My brain couldn't conceive of the idea of being asexual, so I decided to do something to ensure I would still desire lovemaking with another person. At that time, it could have been with either a man or a woman.

According to the dictionary, the word "libido" means:

1. The psychic and emotional energy associated with the instinctual biological drives.
2. Manifestation of sexual drive.
3. Sexual desire.

If there is a psychological component to a person's libido, then couldn't the brain be trained to maintain the same level of libido after a male-to-female transsexual begins hormone treatment? I felt truly motivated to find out the answer to that question.

The physical effects of taking female hormones were not only well documented on the internet and in books, but my friends provided me with their first-hand experiences on this matter. The penis would shrink and no longer feel the same sensations it felt before hormones. That idea didn't bother me, because I would eventually have it inverted for my new vagina. Of course at that time, I didn't think I would live a full decade without getting sex reassignment surgery. If the penis couldn't feel pleasure and I didn't want it to, then where on my body would that pleasure come from?

The first place I concentrated on was my nipples. They had proven to feel sensitivity in the past, so I focused on finding the right way to make them feel it again. In a very short time, I discovered that if I wet the tips of my fingers and very lightly rub them over the tips of my nipples, I would feel some tingling sensation. It took me a while to actually magnify that sensation and "train" my brain to understand that this was a new erogenous zone. It worked.

As satisfying as my nipples felt during that "training period," I knew that there had to be more. This time, I turned my attention a bit further south, a place where my future vagina would reside. I knew that the nerve bundle in the area between the testicles felt some form of sensation, but nothing prepared me for what I would discover when I started concentrating on that area. To say I found my ultimate G-spot would be a gross understatement. Nothing in my life has ever felt that amazing and it didn't take any time for my brain to register this new erogenous zone. I created these new pleasure points before I began taking hormones and my penis had shrunk. Feeling a female-like orgasm without getting an erection made me ecstatic. And, having multiple orgasms opened a whole new world for me. My journey as a female had begun.

In later years, I had a conversation with a therapist who not only worked with transgender people, but with paraplegics and quadriplegics. She would help them find sexual pleasure in the areas where they still had feelings, training the pleasure center of the brain to accept these locations as their new erogenous zones. It appears I had followed her methods before I knew that sort of brain-training existed.

Knowing that I had the ability to enjoy a full and wonderful sex life as a woman–whether I had surgery or not–strengthened my libido rather than diminished it. I looked forward to finding the love of my life rather than shrinking away and avoiding love altogether. It made me less afraid to wear my heart on my sleeve, less afraid to open up to someone and less afraid to have my heart broken.

Just before and after I began living as a woman, I felt a need to experience love with men. I had fantasies of actually living with a man and having a happy home as a married woman later in my life. I quickly discovered that the men who found pre-operative, male-to-female transsexuals exciting looked for just one thing. They want a "chick with a dick" . . . the mystical "Best-of-Both-Worlds" creature. They do indeed exist in the form of she-males, but an MTF transsexual has a different motive for living as a woman. Since taking hormones causes a pre-op, MTF transsexual's penis to shrink and not get erect, then this may turn off many men who want to date a pre-op.

Sex with men felt exciting, but as time went on, I needed more than a quick roll in the sack. My attraction to masculinity faded, replaced completely by the need for the softness and emotional gratification I had always received from women. It meant I really didn't change who I found attractive, so by definition, I went from being a heterosexual man to being a gay woman. Only the labels changed. I now tell people I'm "historically bisexual," since I did have sex with men at one time in my life.

Now that I had finally discovered my true sexual orientation, what would I do next? Fate would place me where I needed to be. In early 2000, I met an attractive, post-operative, MTF transsexual who seemed to find me attractive as well. We met in Phoenix while she attended a political activism meeting I had put on. We hit it off rather quickly and later in the evening, she and I went dancing at the local lesbian club. While on the dance floor, she pulled me close to her and kissed me. My first kiss from a post-op woman and it felt so good that it made me weak at the knees.

Sadly, the evening didn't find us sharing a bed together. She made an odd blanket statement stating that post-op transsexual women do not want to make love to pre-op transsexual women, because it reminds them of their past. To her, it felt like "going back in time." She also said that it makes the pre-op jealous. At that time, I believed her statement was widely accepted by post-op women, but later I found out that her attitude only reflected her own personal feelings and nothing more. Over the past seven years, I've had the pleasure of making love to several post-op women, so I'm now positive not everyone accepts her viewpoint.

My first true love as Monica came only five months after kissing that woman on the dance floor. She, too, was a post-op MTF transsexual, having had her surgery eight years earlier. I met her on a list for trans people, but it didn't have many members from Arizona. The two of us talked on the phone for a while then decided to get together one Saturday to go to a movie. For this story, I will call her Brenda.

Brenda and I hit it off rather well and found out we had at least a few things in common. She told me that for the past twelve years she had been living with a man, but it just didn't feel right to her. Since she began her transition during the days when the doctors insisted a person follow very strict rules, she had to convince them of being straight or they wouldn't let her continue. The doctors wouldn't allow any transsexual to identify as being gay. Many lied to the doctors, some so convincing that they believed it themselves. Thus was the case with Brenda.

I found Brenda attractive, but the words of the other woman five months earlier still rang in my ears. "Post-ops don't want to make love to pre-ops." This meant Brenda and I would be nothing more than friends, which I could easily settle for. However, fate stepped in once again and threw me a most interesting curve ball.

After going to the movies and having lunch together, we came back to my place and began talking about all sorts of things, including our past and how our families treated us. I cannot remember who broached the subject first, but the topic of sex and love came up. Sometime during that subject, she asked me, "Have you ever made love to post-op?"

I said, "I got the impression that post-ops didn't want to have anything to do with pre-ops."

Brenda found that statement to be completely ridiculous. To prove it, she leaned in close and gave me a long and sensual kiss. Wow. What made me so lucky to get kissed by such a gorgeous woman? They say that what comes around goes around. Whatever I did to deserve such good karma, I needed to keep doing it.

After some extensive foreplay, Brenda and I ended up in bed together. I've had memorable times making love to another person, but that first night with Brenda topped anything I had ever experienced up until then. (But, my future had better things in store for me in later years.) She solidified my sexual orientation. From that evening on, I would never consider making love to a man—except a trans man. Why, you may ask? Trans men have a quality about them that nontrans men don't. Some will admit it, while others won't. Their past gives them a much deeper appreciation for women, so they know how to treat a woman right—at least most of them do.

Over the next few weeks, Brenda and I had fantastic nights together; nights that burn deep into my memory with the passion we felt for each other. However, life would not allow us to continue our relationship. Just before I met Brenda, I had applied for another job in Atlanta, staying within the company I worked for. They accepted me and asked me to arrive in Atlanta by June 12, 2000. I had to leave just as our relationship began to heat up. She and I remained friends for a few years after I left, but as of today, she won't take any of my calls. I would like to find out if she has a happy life.

My life in Georgia was totally different than what I experienced in Arizona. The people at my new job accepted me completely and I had more challenges on the job than I did in Phoenix. Other opportunities opened up to me as a political activist, putting me in a position to meet many people in the area and nationwide. My experience with women didn't take off until I had been there for about five months. "Five months?" Again? Is this a reoccurring pattern? I wonder. . .? Transgender people are great with trigonometry, because they love to go off on tangents.

Where was I? Oh, yes. Five months after I arrived in Georgia, I met another post-op transsexual at Atlanta's first Transgender Day of Remembrance. I will call her Olivia. Something about her caught my eye. I felt drawn to her looks and intelligence. What can I say? I find highly intelligent women very sexy and Olivia fit the bill on that, as Brenda had earlier. For the next two months, we had a torrid relationship. The fact that she lived in Athens, about 90 miles away from where I lived at the time, caused a bit of a problem for me. Getting there took up a lot of my time and gas.

Even though everything seemed to be going smoothly between the two of us, Olivia had something boiling deep in the bowels of her psyche. She had a dark past of disturbing incidents that had left her emotionally and psychologically scarred. Many transsexuals experience horrible things in their life and none of them make it through unscathed. Some are harmed far more than others. Olivia carried the wounds of family rejection and physical and mental abuse that stayed hidden just below the surface like an emotional Mt. St. Helen, waiting for the right—or wrong—moment to erupt. That eruption took place about two months into our relationship.

On the day it happened, I stayed over night at Olivia's apartment. The next day she seemed all lovey-dovey when we got up and we planned on seeing a movie that afternoon. Before the movie, I stopped at an eyeglass store to get new glasses and she wandered through the mall. After I finished getting everything ordered, I waited and waited for her to come back. When she did, she seemed distant and didn't want to talk. We went to the movie and during the entire time, she leaned away from me, not making any physical contact.

On the drive home, she remained silent. I knew then that she wanted to break up with me. I asked, "Is it over?"

"Wait until we get back to my place."

I started crying. She showed no emotion. The pain cut through my heart.

When we arrived at her place, she turned to me and in the coldest tone of voice, she said, "I want you to leave."

"Why? What happened? We were okay just this morning."

She said nothing and still showed no emotions. It appeared to me that this post-op transsexual shifted into a mode that I hadn't ever seen in a woman, breaking up with me like any man would break up with a woman. I felt like an emotional basket case on that long drive home.

In later years, Olivia told me she shouldn't have let me go. My friends and I later found out that Olivia led a transient life, not wanting to get a job and had tried to con others into giving her money. I also found out just recently that she now lives in San Francisco and has been stalking a prominent facial surgeon, trying to get him to do surgery on her for free. Olivia has even tried to commit suicide several times. She really needs help.

Losing Olivia when I did couldn't have happened at a better time. Not only did I dodge the bullet with her early on in the relationship, but it freed me to begin looking elsewhere. A couple of weeks later, I attended a Georgia Stonewall Democrats meeting and I told a female friend of mine, Sara, about how Olivia had treated me. Sara asked, "Does this mean I can now ask you out on a date?"

"Ah . . . ah, yes. It does."

I found Sara to be not only highly intelligent, but she and I had several things in common. We both love science fiction and we both love to write, though her writing focuses on nonfiction, whereas I have a love for fiction. In school, Sara considered herself a computer geek and looking back at myself in school, I was a nerd. At the time I met her, she worked as an editor for a trade magazine, but had also written for the local GLBT newspaper and wrote for CNN.

On our first date, I took her to an Italian restaurant and we talked about several things. I found her attractive and felt comfortable being with her. That evening, we went back to my place and made love on the couch in the living room. Wrong move.

My roommate, another transsexual and owner of the townhouse I lived in, confronted me the next day and ordered me to move out in six months. She never said why she gave me so much time, but I figured she needed extra money to help pay for her upcoming labiaplasty. I discovered later that the whole reason she needed me to move in was to help her get the final amount of money she needed for her sex reassignment surgery. Once my usefulness had ended, I would be kicked out anyway. My evening with Sara accelerated that. The next day, I began looking for a place and found one much closer to work and to Sara. My former roommate would have to find her money somewhere else.

Sara and I had an interesting relationship. For four years, we called each other "girlfriends," using the lesbian definition and not the one used by straight women when referring to their female friends. We expressed our love for each other in many ways, but we never had a sex life after that first date. I found out she had a bipolar condition and because of the medicines she had to take, she completely lost her libido. Of course, my libido remained as strong as ever during the entire relationship.

I once asked Sara, "Do you find any woman on earth sexually attractive?" She responded by saying "No." If Sara felt that way about every woman, then I didn't have much of a problem with our lack of sex life, at least at first. It became clear to me as time went on that it had become a growing problem. She encouraged me to seek out others for sex, but I only found someone twice in the entire four years. Later, her doctor gave her a new drug that helped to restore her libido, but it became quickly apparent that she still didn't want to make love with me, even when her libido returned. It became the start of our downhill slide. As time went on, other things contributed to our eventual breakup. We kept growing apart until my lack of enthusiasm forced her to call it quits. The moment of our breakup felt sad, but necessary to give me a chance to grow and expand. My relationship with Sara did me a lot of good and helped me to further understand myself in many ways that I couldn't have if she and I had never dated. We remain friends to this day.

In April of 2005, I met a woman, Cissy, at a local lesbian nightclub called My Sister Room (MSR). Since this nightclub sat across the tracks from the all-women college, Agnes Scott, it drew in a lot of women in their early twenties. I could easily tell that Cissy didn't fit that age bracket because of her gray hair.

Cissy and I stayed together for a few months, even though she never felt comfortable seeing me completely nude. I had to hide my penis by wearing panties, yet she didn't mind eventually being totally nude with me. She wouldn't allow me to give her oral sex, so we had to use other ways to take care of her needs. However, she spent very little time taking care of my needs.

Because Cissy lived forty miles away and didn't have transportation, it became hard on me. Also, she shared her house with a much older woman whose attitude forced Cissy to not invite friends over without causing a big fuss. I had to drive to Cissy's place, bring her back to my apartment so we could go out or have dinner together, then drive her home the next day. This became too much after a while, so I broke it off with her.

The week after I broke it off with Cissy, I met another woman at MSR. This time I went there to just enjoy myself and not to try to hook up with someone. But, hook up I did, and in a huge way. The woman I met that night, Gina, had something about her that I found intriguing. Normally, I'm attracted to femme women, but Cissy and Gina didn't fit that category one bit. However, I found Gina very attractive and interesting to talk to. She works as a lawyer for a firm that helps to patent biotech creations for companies. This job was tailor-made for her, since she has a degree in both biology and law.

After we left MSR, we grabbed a bite to eat at an all-night diner, then she took me to her place. The fact that she didn't care about my "plumbing irregularities" surprised and thrilled me, since I told her well in advance about me, back at MSR. Her lack of shyness felt refreshing after my experiences with Sara and Cissy.

That evening began a five-month relationship that rivaled anything else in my entire life. (Again, with the "five-months"?) Our lovemaking took me to a new level of ecstasy that I never believed existed and I had only heard rumors of over the years. I place the stories of that kind of intense lovemaking in the same category as ghosts, angels, and UFOs. I've heard of them, but I never personally encountered them. We did things together that I would have never expected from any woman. I fell in love once again, only this time in a hard way.

Gina had separated from a woman whom she had a committed relationship with just six months earlier. She was the biological mother of a five-year-old girl and shared joint custody with her ex. One weekend Gina would have the girl and the next weekend her ex would, so we "hooked up" on those weekends when she didn't have her daughter. However, we would go to dinner and do things together on the weekends she had her daughter.

During the course of our relationship, Gina told me that she had a repressed sex life since her early years and after separating from her ex, she had finally liberated herself to explore the hidden desires within. Since we went on that exploration together, uncovering the various facets of her sexual desires, I told her that we were like Lewis and Clark heading up the Missouri river into the mountains, finding new wonders around every bend. I couldn't believe the beauties of what we found along the way. Thinking of those nights still makes me smile.

One of the most touching moments of our relationship took place on Christmas Eve and Christmas morning, 2005. Gina's daughter asked if I could "sleep over" that night so I could spend Christmas morning with them. Gina agreed. I fully expected to sleep in a spare bedroom, but I ended up in Gina's bed. I made sure I had a complete pair of pajamas on, because I felt a bit apprehensive about her daughter being there and possibly wandering into the room. It all turned out fine.

The next morning, I once again experienced the wonder of Christmas through the eyes of a small child, something I hadn't felt since the early 1990s. No other Christmas during the entire time living as Monica felt as wonderful. I would have pledged my commitment to Gina that very morning if she had asked me.

One funny thing happened at Christmas that still makes me laugh when I think about it. Gina's daughter received a little girl's make-up kit as one of her gifts. After opening it, she turned to Gina and asked if she could help in putting on the make-up. Gina laughed and said she was the last person to ask on how to properly apply makeup. Monica to the rescue! I piped up and said, "Well, it looks like this is an area I'm familiar with. Let me help you." Gina's daughter was excited. While Gina made breakfast in the kitchen, I showed her daughter the proper way to put on make-up. Since I had two sons, I never felt the joy of helping a young girl apply make-up properly.

What factored heavily into why Gina and I had a short relationship had to be the "rebound syndrome." Even though we had a short-lived and intense romance, we ended it as very close friends. She has become one of the few people I know who I can confide in with the most intimate details of my life. We stay in touch and have breakfast or dinner together occasionally, along with her daughter. When my mother came to visit me for a week in April, the four of us went to the new Georgia Aquarium together. My mother had nothing but high praise for Gina.

I haven't had a steady girlfriend since Gina and I broke up, but I've had some rather interesting romantic moments during that time. In late September, when the Southern Comfort Conference took place in Atlanta, many of my friends from across the country attended. I had the chance to make love to two trans women at the same time, one post-op and one pre-op. It may sound exciting, but part of the evening, the other two spent a very long time concentrating on each other. I even got up and got dressed before they noticed I was in the room. And yet, I suggested having the threesome in the first place. I thought that if I would ever have the fortune of being with two women at the same time, each of us would be treated with equality. I may not suggest threesomes in the future.

I did learn one thing during that encounter. I quickly found out that the pre-op had the same erogenous zones as I have. Very interesting. Once I discovered this, I wouldn't stop until she begged me to. I can easily say she enjoyed herself, as did I.

During that Southern Comfort Conference, I did something else exciting and new. I asked a good friend of mine, a professional photographer, to take nude photos of me, in black and white. She took nearly two rolls of pictures that day and in some of the photos, someone else was there with me. As I write this piece, I haven't seen the pictures, but the other person in them with me has. She said they turned out great.

After reading this, one might think that I've had a rather exciting sex life with all the women I've met. Yet, I finish this piece with nothing more than a sigh to comfort me. Like I said, I don't have that one special person to share my life with at this time. No one is near me, reading over my shoulder, begging me to save what I have typed and come to bed. Do I want someone? Yes. Will I stop after getting my heart broken again and again? Never! If I did, the next person I would have met could have been "The One," so I continue to move forward.

My life has had many moments of sheer pleasure and beauty, sur-rounded with mundane days, weeks, and even months. But, I'm en-couraged that fate has more interesting moments ahead. And who knows, maybe the next time transgender people are asked to submit a story about how love works with them, I will be able to write an ex-tensive piece about my lifelong love. Until then, I will have to be sat-isfied with the cards life has dealt me.

13

Between Shows: A True Story

Lee "Bridgett" Harrington

OPENING SHOW

I'd been working my ass off all day. There are worse jobs to have than globe-trotting as an erotic educator, teaching swingers, perverts, and your average college kids how to have a better sex life and tie each other up in bed. But after five hours of teaching in one afternoon, and after having flown fourteen hours the day before from the U.S. to Australia, I was wiped out.

Sadly, wiped out was not an option. I had agreed to fly from Melbourne to Sydney after my classes were done to perform at one of the most notorious parties in the scene down under—No Holes Barred. Run by Ultra, the hostess who organizes monthly fetish night Hellfire, No Holes Barred takes place in abandoned warehouse spaces whenever Ultra feels randomly inspired. These spaces get transformed by a team of sweaty leather men and women into a den of debauchery. As I showed up at the venue hauling a bag of rope, wardrobe, high heels, and trailing behind a great entourage of friends I'd met stateside who'd convinced me to come to the land down under, I was struck by how much transformation had taken place.

As you passed through giant velvet labia, the huge room had been transformed into a dark and dingy dance floor, the perfect quantities of seedy sexuality and open rave space, with an upstairs balcony looking down on the dancers. Then off to the right they'd turned another pair of rooms into dungeon spaces where the denizens who had such desires could wield their whips and wicked words. Back outside, under an early Australian fall clear night sky, they had set up couches, chairs, benches, two bars, a stage show area, and cloakrooms. Already, only thirty minutes into festivities, the couches were already full of scantily-clad lesbians, hot fags, gaggles of swinging het folk involved in deep conversation, and the occasional heavy petting. If someone had told me that I'd find the man of my dreams there, I would have laughed. I'm still laughing.

I dropped off my bag in the cloakroom and got to the business of getting dressed. Unlike many other venues I've done performance art at, No Holes Barred was distinctly lacking in dressing rooms. I've done worse things than change in public though, so I went to business wriggling into opera-length baby pink seamed stockings, platform open-toed heels, a pink and black girdle, black lacy bra and knickers, and hyper-femme make-up.

Dressing up like this is almost always a mixed-emotion experience for me. As a male-identified, female-bodied individual, it's sometimes hard to draw the line between feeling sexy as a biologically gifted drag queen and a tormented man screaming to get away from the longing looks from Kinsey six lesbians and open-ended offers from heterosexual male swingers hoping to hook up for the night. I love the sensation of finely woven silk sliding against my silky legs, of my girdle or corset cinching down around my waist, of my lipstick lacquering my lips with crimson courage. It is delicious to feel the longing as I'm stared at from hundreds of hungry eyes—but then it snaps back and I realize what they are lusting after is not what I am. Which is why, when he got his words back later that night, I melted. When he told me that the drag I'd been wearing earlier looked fucking amazing on me. It's hard to find people who get that it is just that—drag—and I knew from those words that this was the kind of guy I could fall for. I fell hard. Good thing that by then I'd changed out of the heels.

I found my performance partner, a hot Italian man with enough machismo for three, and we headed off to get ready. We set up on the outside suspension rig having watched the piercing performance artists finish up their work, and started throwing rope. For each rope he threw, I threw one of my own, weaving me in an intricate web of hemp lines around my lingerie clad form. Slowly the crowd around us started to grow as he hoisted me up into the air and spread my legs wide. I laughed and moaned as he pulled me up to him and worked a glove hand first into my hungry mouth and then into whatever orifice he could find. We'd promised the folks at No Holes a show to remember, and as the cum flew, leaving pools beneath me, we certainly delivered.

Later I found out he'd only caught part of the show. So be it. It wasn't the shows that mattered. It was knowing that those two shows stood like book ends over the first two weeks of our romance.

After I was mopped up from the stage, I realized that the air had grown crisp so I went back to the cloakroom and slipped off the heels and replaced them with heavy sixteen-inch Carolina logging boots. The seamed stockings and girdle stayed, but I added a heavier jacket and went back out to brave the crowd. Smiles, introductions, kisses, and lovely banter filled the next half an hour, until the monotony of hiding behind a wall of pretty women got to me and I went back out into the party.

My ears caught onto the familiar sound of a west coast American accent, and I followed it to its source. Sitting on a bench outside was a delicious poster boy for leather fetishism—a tall, dark-haired creamy-skinned man with flat abs clad head to toe in biker garb that he looked like he'd been poured into. He was having his boots polished and worshipped by a big bear of a man, dark blue mohawk, and hands dark with polish, as I asked if I could join him. "Please!" It's such a pleasure to hear a familiar accent. I laughed and knew we'd get along grand.

It turned out that this leather god before me was a friend of a friend from the Bay Area in California, and as he told me details of his life and joys of the Sydney scene, my attention kept drifting off towards the boot slut at his feet. Many years ago in New York my friend Jim turned me onto the sensual delight that is having your boots done by a boot slut while still laced into them, and I had never forgotten—and this boy down on the concrete certainly knew his way around a pair. I looked down at my own Carolinas and realized just how poor of a shape they were in, and became determined that I would find someone to do them for me that night.

After saying farewell and petting the boot pup on his head, I wandered off to find the other boot black I'd seen that night. A tiny trans man in overalls had been going around proclaiming how he wasn't allowed to wear leather until he'd blacked 100 pairs of boots according to his lover, and I wanted to help him out. I tried and tried, but no luck;

the sweet young thing had simply vanished so I grabbed a drink instead.

I sat down with the women I knew, and a few minutes later the boot pup I'd seen at the leather god's feet was wandering by. Good, finally a chance to look at him. He stood about 5'7" with big tattoos on his muscled forearms, one of a wolf and the twin towers, and the other of a pair of Tom of Finland boys locked in a passionate embrace. He was wearing dark trousers and a top, with a tool belt slung around his hips full of all manner of polishing gear for indulging in his fetish. At the base of the look was a pair of immaculately kept black leather boots that shone out like polished stones against the gray asphalt beneath us. He smirked slightly as I called him over with a motion of my hand.

The Bear turned towards me and it hit me then that I had no idea what gender he was. I knew he was a he because he exuded masculinity, from his subtle signs of submission to his cocky little grin. I knew he was a he because of the way he kissed my hand like only guys do— butch dykes who use "she" rarely get it quite right. I knew he was a he because he made my inner cock jump alive in the way that only gay boys, specifically Bears, do.

It didn't matter though, did it? What mattered was finding out his name and whether he'd be interested in doing my boots. Parker introduced himself (odd now to remember our old names, since his name changed to Hank and mine changed to Lee), and said he would be happy to be of service. My heart fluttered at realizing that just like the gender issue, I had no idea who was on "top" in this power dynamic. Was he playing me like a fiddle and seducing the femme just to get his hands on hir, or was I seeing a submissive blossom beneath my touch? It didn't matter though, did it?

As he offered out his hand, lines of polish dug in beneath his nails to my immaculate paw with polished tips that matched my lips, I realized how tall I must seem next to him. I was better than before, where my platform heels had made me stand almost 6'3," but even being almost six foot tall in my heavy leather boots was daunting for most. He didn't seem to care though. He walked just as tall, not puffing himself up like a big fish like so many men do next to the leggy dames. He pulled me up a chair and seemed to me as large as the universe itself. And then he let me sit, and suddenly I was transformed into the queen of that universe.

Queen being the primary word here. I in no way felt like a woman around him, and the energy flying between our lingering gazes was that of two hot men who understood butch/femme dynamics are not just for the girls. He turned around after chucking his head sideways at me for a moment, as if he'd seen it too but was confused. I then realized that this big thug of a man before me had someone in service to him standing six feet away, and he ordered her to grab a few extra supplies for him.

If I hadn't been in lust before, I was now. As a person who himself enjoys both sides of power dynamics, both sides of gender expression, both sides of sadism and masochism, I have a soft spot for other people who find grace on both sides of the fence. We are not fence sitters, we are people who have a key to the gate between. And as I saw Parker turn from his Alpha Girl back towards me and sink back into his sensual act of seductive submission, he had me.

He knelt at my boots and slowly unlaced the first, laying the worn cord around his neck like an open tie. His green-gray eyes looked up at me on occasion from his work but for the most part he focused on my worn boots. These boots have seen me across five continents, attended desert raves and hiked through snow storms, have had their soles replaced twice and still their soul is intact. Parker understood this as I told the tales of the leather between his fingertips and he caressed the worn hide like a lover who was overdue for a massage.

For each boot he worked in a linear process, from cleaning with saddle soap to applying polish with his finger tips. He'd then move on to rubbing the polish in with the broad flat of his meaty hands as I imagined those hands balling up into fists and making their way inside of me. Worked in, he pulled out a brush and rubbed with delicious speed and simultaneous tenderness. He then turned to his kit and realized he didn't have any pantyhose to develop a high shine . . . this is where the femme gets to pull out the stops.

"Oh, do you need some?" I asked, and slowly slipped my foot out of the half-done boot. I undid the garters at the top of the seamed stocking, lifted my leg high above his head, and with impossible slowness slid the pink mesh down off of my leg. Resting down at my ankles, I grabbed the toe of the stocking and pulled on it, creating this long stream of silk flying off my now bare and smooth leg and up into the air. His jaw almost dropped as I offered it to him saying only, "It had a rip in it, see? It might as well go to good use."

Even if it had had no run in it, I would have torn it just to be able to pull off that reaction. These are the dirty tricks we femmes keep hidden up our sleeves.

He accepted the offering like a holy item. Coveting it for a moment, I could tell he was feeling my heat off of the silk, imagining his own body pressed against that heat, but then he went back to work. Silk flew against leather at a dizzying rate until a high shine shone back from my old friend on my foot, and he turned his attention to my other boot after lacing back up the first. Laces out, saddle soap, polish with fingers, worked in with a brush, and again the silk danced in the air as pink gossamer turned tarnished under his fingers and I showed him a few tricks with blacking he hadn't seen before.

He could serve, but could he play? I had to know, and soon I knew. He could. But that involved leaving the stage area of the opening show.

SECOND SHOW

Hellfire Sydney is known for its dark den of decadence, where the highest in fetish fashion mixes with the raw hedonism of sensuality while wild stage shows and hard beats light up the dance floor. I had been invited to be one of those wild stage shows. Having Parker at my call, first I asked if he'd be willing to be my cohort on stage, then I asked if he knew of anyone perfect for my plans. My initial model wasn't quite hardcore enough for my desired show, and he knew just the perfect soul for my staged sacrifice.

The model he'd had in mind was a body modification fanatic named Zoo. Zoo was slender, big-breasted, and had a huge tattoo on her hip labeling her as Grade A meat. Her facial piercings were not distracting from her academic punk beauty, and her black hair framed her face perfectly. Add to this the fact that Zoo loved being physically challenged, and it was a perfect match. Parker certainly did know his stuff. The show was a simple plan—demon waits on stage while second demon hauls in a fighting virgin to be sacrificed. It's been done a thousand times. But we had a few twists of drama waiting.

Backstage I looked into the mirror, then back at Parker. We'd spent almost two whole weeks effectively glued to each other, and the rate at which we were predicting each other was getting creepy, but in a good way. He handed me the red make-up as I transformed him from a brutal Bear into a demonic thug, gluing his horns to his head and adding detailing around his eyes and mouth. We traded spaces and I turned into the mirror and did my own make-up, with a heavy red horizontal band across my eyes accentuated by glitter and black eyeliner to make my white eye contacts pop under the stage lights. We turned to Zoo and said, "No make-up, no shoes, no underwear." Just a simple sheet we could cut off if we so chose.

Parker was dressed in his Los Angeles Police Department uniform, dark and menacing, while I wriggled into a slightly more complicated costume. Fake fur trousers with an attached tail went on first, followed by a black sequined bra, see-through black and silver mesh top, then on went the boots with Parker down at my feet to do the buckles. These platform knee-high boots looked more like hooves wrapped in buckles, and with each stomp on the ground I could energetically feel the earth shake beneath me. Then on went a black leather underbust corset that I was laced tightly into, and locked the buckles up the center of the cincher down with nimble fingers. Finally I put a huge piece of amber around my neck, and we were ready to go.

As the dancers began to clear, I cued the DJ. "My Sacrifice" crept into the audio track of 300 hungry minds as they took seats or gathered around as Zoo's sudden scream broke them from their trance. I locked eyes with Parker and he brought the screaming girl in his arms over to me as I licked my lips underneath the metal frame. Blue hemp rope flew over white flesh and with a single long length I had her arms and chest bound and she was tied off to the frame as she squirmed in time with the music. Out came needles to be pushed through her flesh, then more rope as I hauled her into the air like the meat she labeled herself as.

The show danced on that way, with needles removed and blood flowing as we demons molested her on stage just as we'd prearranged. Finally, we lowered her to the ground and I let out a roar to clear the path as my thug Bear carried the breathing maiden carcass over his shoulder and off to the dressing room.

Between our sweat and a lack of any air conditioning, the dressing room, which was in fact just the disabled toilet with a lock on it, was unbearably hot. My fake fur clung to me and I needed desperately to get out of my leather as well. My boy went to unbuckling my boots as I ripped madly at my corset, hoping to be free. The show had been great, but there had been a plan for other blood play, between Parker and I, on stage. It hadn't happened, and he and I both knew it. We ripped at my clothes and everything went flying.

Finally down to nothing but my make-up and skin, Parker grabbed a hold of me. He handed me a bottle of water and made me sit down on the toilet. Breathe. Breathe for me baby. Come on, don't freak out on me. I downed the water bottle in one gulp and threw it to the side. I was dehydrated, drained, and overheated. Badly overheated. But mostly I was drained emotionally. And Parker knew what to do. I'd told him, shown him, and in two swift weeks he'd learned ways to calm me down. I get so worked up sometimes, so manic—had it only been two weeks?

BETWEEN SHOWS

Two days after the first show, I had gone to meet my friend Cub to go snorkeling. He asked me at the stairs of the train station, "Do you mind that I brought someone?" We climbed up the stairs, and there he was wearing a U.S. Marine Corp cap. Cub, you dirty bastard, I love you.

That day was too cold to go snorkeling as planned, so we headed out to Manly Bay across the water from downtown Sydney by boat. The ferry ride was perfect. The three of us trannybears (ok, I'm just a furless cub) were a perfect team, Cub and I splashing in the water with the fish while Parker watched our bags, and then the whole trio of us burying our bliss into ribs and steaks. Parker told me he'd stalked me online. I told him he hit thirty of my buttons in one quick story. We all laughed, and inside I melted even more.

Later that night after a frantic run around of getting flyers out for my classes due to clerical errors, I turned around in the car my friend was driving and asked Parker if he had a curfew. He looked at me, baffled. After two minutes of me trying to be subtle, Jo turned around and said, "Honey, you're being asked if you want to come back to our place." His eyes almost fell out of his head as the big intelligent brute of a man I'd spent the day with transformed into a wide-eyed puppy wanting to wag his tail.

He attended my art show opening. He came to my drag king and strip show. He led the advertising for my meet and greet. He demo bottomed for two of my classes that next weekend. He cheered me on as I read three of my pieces at the spoken word night. But more importantly than any of those things was the fact that he let me cry. He let me scream. He let me moan and open my soul wide as a river's mouth as I ushered him into my heart. And he told me his tale; a tale of gender and sex, a tale of pain and pleasure, a tale of bodies still not matching truths—and I understood his pain. His pain was mine. And we cried together.

Between shows he accepted the offer of my working collar, a ring through his nose, a sign of testing a formality of service and structured relationship. He never doubted to call me Sir. Even as my high heels locked around the back of his neck, he looked in my eyes and he got it, because he could see me inside the biologically gifted drag queen shell.

Amazing things can happen between shows. Just as ten minutes on stage can play out the tale of a virgin's suffering in hell for eternity, just as a hedonistic exhibit of delights dances on for ages when only fifteen minutes have passed according to the clock, so too can two weeks transform into a lifetime. We wrote in two weeks more tales than many dare to live in a lifetime because we dared. Because we saw each other as the men we were, the men we are, offstage, between shows.

14

To the Three Women I Loved in My Transgender Life

TinyBelly

A TURNING POINT

I retraced the conversation records, looking at those arguments with you, so that I can't suppress my complex tempers to compare them with our friend-like relationship now.

That day, on the feminism course, we sat together by chance. I shared my lecture handouts with you and this became the beginning of our familiarity. You were a lesbian; I was a male to female transgender—even though you didn't know anything about this, just taking me to be a typical girl.

You were not only smart, but strong-minded. Every time we met, the topics were either science and philosophy, or feminism; it benefited each of us a lot in the communion of knowledge. When we ambled around the campus in the night, letting the cold-white streetlight spray on our bodies, you asked, "So you were studying in Tainan Girls' Senior High School?"

"No," I replied. Having studied at the boys' high school, I trembled with fear, fearing so deeply of having to come out without any preparation in mind, and that you would be close to me no more. As a matter of fact, deep inside my heart, the thirst for intimacy brought me a gleam of hope, but I also did not have any expectation for further intimacy—my biological sex is male, I had not yet had sex reassignment surgery and you are a femme—how can we have any possibilities to make advances?

Trans People In Love

"I was actually often afraid—deeply afraid—that everything is an illusion . . . I felt I seem to navigate a boat in a storm, and the helm has to be controlled so hardily," you said to me on the Internet.

Yes, I knew your feelings, but I couldn't ignore the male flesh and express my appreciation to you—that would be like I was cheating; the great worry of our friendship being broken made me stop in my tracks before coming out. Slowly, heavily, and anxiously, I typed, "I'm a male to female transgender," on the screen. I couldn't, and didn't want to keep this disguise on in front of you anymore. It was just like the TV shows: a friend you knew so well or the one who used to sleep with you told you suddenly that she was not the sex you thought—so shocking.

"I'm really so lucky to know you," you replied and did not change your behavior towards me; I was excited and blissful. I didn't think there was any probability of me entering any intimate relationships.

That same night during which the dialogue occurred, you and I were in different cities. The thing was that I, the one who was bathing in pleasure, did not know that you, in Taipei city, sitting opposite a friend who'd joined you for a night snack, cried out loud: "How could this thing happen? She is a man . . ."

The next evening, you and I met on the Net again. You did not change your mind, just as yesterday, choosing to give us a try; I burst into tears because of being touched deep in my soul. After confirming our feelings to each other, this day became my first red-letter day, indicating love in my life.

You and I made an attempt to have one of those so-called open relationships because we didn't want to link absolutely a partner relationship and having sex together. As a result, I did not have sex with any others from the beginning to the end of our relationship; and you had only one time making love with a butch. Even until this day, I find it was an interesting memory in my life sharing your "unfaithful" experience.

I felt so sorry that when I brought you south you could not help attending the meals my relatives invited you to because they wanted to take a look at you since you were my girlfriend and I was still a man because I had not come out to all the members of my family. A simple trip thus became an interview with a quasi-daughter-in-law and this limited the time we had to make tours around my home city. You said that as a lesbian, this also gave you many tastes and experiences that you had never had and would not have.

As for your family, the situation was quite different. It took eight years for your mother to accept that you were a lesbian. In order not to add too many burdens to her heart, I was scrupulous about everything each time I went to your house for fear of her noticing that your new girlfriend was a biological man; however, one year passed away rapidly and nothing happened.

You brought me many "first times:" first intimate relationship, first time having self-confidence in my appearance, first person to let me know my weakness inside. You were also the first one to see my male and female side at the same time. At school and with family, I used the male appearance expected by others, but while with friends or outside, I would appear as female. There was one time my father telephoned me while we were strolling around the Shi-Lin night market. I was very ambivalent about whether I should answer the phone. After all, you certainly would hear/see my behavior as a male. Finally, I felt easy and pushed the answer button after you said it's ok. But somehow, this made you have a stomachache for a long time.

You went window shopping with me, taught me tricks about wearing clothes, listened to my never-ending complaints about my body, joined in trans celebrations, such as the Transgender Rainbow Party with me, saw me practicing the bunny girls' dance for the Sex Workers Culture Festival, gave me courage so that I could brace myself for gradually being me, made me self-confident, instead of being drawn deep into the sorrow of being the wrong sex, provided me with opportunities to enter women's culture, thus helping me to start to learn about being a woman, and taught me what love was.

In that period, habitual loneliness had caused me, a freshman in the field of love, and having been used to living a single lifestyle, to see things solely from my point of view and to show no consideration for you; therefore you, the one who had such rich experiences with relationships, were extraordinarily tired out and we had innumerable arguments. The only image I had at the beginning of our relationship was that of you leaving out of anger.

One night filled with coldness, you came back to Jungli from Taipei to see me. I was using the computer, writing what I wanted to say to you, but not considering pouring a cup of warm water for you. It was the middle of the night, one of many. I forget the details but you left my house in a bad mood. A more serious argument took place on Christmas Eve. Because of my careless fault, you took the bus right after leaving the house and refused to contact me or see me for two full weeks when you arrived in Taipei.

Afterwards, as I learned to correct my faults, our relationship slowly became harmonious; however, on the sex side, you and I were not really compatible. The quality of our sex was quite good though, although it was difficult to come to a satisfying conclusion on how often we should do it. My desire was lower than yours, so that led to you being unfulfilled quite a lot of the time. One night, you and I argued over our sex life as usual; you sat smoking at the table, angry. You looked at me as I lay on the bed sobbing, then you left me in your house and rode out on your motorcycle to find a person to talk to. These things challenged the affections between us. Suffering an education for being a man and learning to hide what was inside my heart for more than twenty years, I became a robot who could not feel his/her feelings, and this enhanced the emotional gap between us.

In the end, we failed to maintain our relationship. On the way to campus, I suggested that we break up. You often mentioned the problems we had before, but I did not have the ability to deal with them. Even though I still had affections towards you, my disability let me realize that they could not be solved in a short while. I could just hope the new distance between you and me could keep our feelings from being spoiled further. Being friends was better than nothing.

THE PASSION

I knew her from the gender and sexuality conference known as the Super-Slim Conference. I had even seen her before in the gay parade, but she didn't know me. At coffee break, she came to say hello, accompanying my friend Rania. I was so shy that I hid myself behind my ex-girlfriend and peeped at her. It was our first contact; later on we discovered that each of us was strongly attracted by the other's temperament just during our first eye contact. Not too long afterwards, we met unexpectedly at the presentation by U.S. trans man, Jamison Green, at the Immigration Assembly Hall. After that I started to have chats with her on the Internet.

She was a queen in SM, not only sunny but also having an affable character. She and I actually had many mutual friends, but had not known each other before. When the friends who knew me and her separately in different places, different times, and different groups found that we got together, they nearly jumped out of their skin. The lesbian, gay, bisexual, transgender, queer (LBGTQ) community was really very small.

She and I fell in love at first sight. Quickly, on New Year's Eve she showed her love to me with a bouquet in the room full of balloons and whispers of love as a beginning of our relationship.

She was a member of Taiwan's bondage/domination/sado-masochism (BDSM) group. I myself was not a BDSM practitioner and neither had we tried SM sex together. At the most, I would lend my body to her to practice on before her rope bondage performance. No matter what, I had more understanding towards BDSM due to her. "I almost didn't make love with a male masochist. We are not lovers, but have an unequal relationship agreed by each other . . . I seldom do SM with a woman because I think she's my girlfriend, not a masochist; "we treat each other equally," she said in an interview with the mass media.

She is a thoughtless and loud person. I, on the other hand, am expressionless, speak little, and always look depressed. We often joked that she and I were just like the combination of an autistic disorder patient and an attention-deficit hyperactivity disorder patient. When two persons with totally different personalities meet together, sometimes they get "neutralization" with no more extremeness. Our differences also produced tension, like an extremely stretched string and we did not know when it would exceed its limits and break. She thought me stony, not uttering endearments, and not showing my yearning for her, even after a long time of separation. I often felt worried about her negligence, which resulted in complaints or distrust.

This year, the first, and up to now, only Asian Lesbian Film and Video Festival in Taiwan was held. She and I went to the Image Museum of Hsinchu Culture to see the movies. There were some of our friends there. When she talked to a not-so-familiar friend, she excitedly mentioned our future plans for our life together. I got extremely worried at that moment in case she was going to accidentally expose my gender identification, so I covered her mouth up with my hands; it was really a bit rude when I look back on it.

Moving to the corner near the wall, she got very angry and thought that I distrusted her. "How is it possible for me to be so stupid that I will speak about it without any considerations?" she queried. Honestly, I had no confidence about it at that time.

In the summer, I told my family about my decision to have sex reassignment surgery. What followed was a complicated mixture of endless tears and anger. She accompanied me when I went back to Tainai to have a chat with my parents. At the coffee shop, my mother wept all the time. "You will undoubtedly regret it if you have surgery! You look like a man; how is it possible for you to become a woman?"

"She is always taken as a female as well as living as one happily; this is what she wants," she replied for me.

"What a silly person! He doesn't regret it because of having not done it! It will be too late to regret if he does it! Do you understand? How silly you are?" my mother said.

It was pretty significant for her to express her opinions as a partner to my surgery. Our society is extremely unimaginative when it comes to people not marrying or to marriages beyond the standard of a male and female; they can never realize and are incapable of believing why a woman, as a male's girlfriend, will take the risk of being unable to marry to support her lover proceeding with TG/TS surgery, and this is why the voices of trans people's partners are important.

After saying goodbye to my mother, we went to the airport to catch a plane to the north. Then she said: "I've got something to tell you . . ."

"What's that?" I asked.

". . . I've fallen in love with my paramour." I listened calmly and then held her in my arms.

She and I tried to have an open relationship. Since we could not meet frequently, and she got frightened easily and felt lonely a lot of the time, she asked me if she could find someone on the Net to keep her company and take her loneliness away. Hence, she had a so-called adulterous partner. "I'll be careful keeping my distance from her. I'll not love her," she said, with confidence at first.

What I failed to consider was that human emotions are not things that can be guaranteed. Our foundations of affections and dependence were not broad-based enough since we had not been together long. She lived near her paramour, so they could meet quite frequently; she and I met each other once a week at most. When it went for longer periods, she was used to doing things with her paramour, and the cords of love between them somehow exceeded ours.

We did not chat much on the plane. "So have we broken up?" I inquired on the streets of Taipei.

"Yes, I think so," she said.

We went to the subway station. This is the place that labeled the end point of our love. I stepped into the carriage, turned my head back, and saw her waving farewell to me. She stood still, following me with her eyes until the train left her vision. I cried out suddenly, with tears flowing uncontrollably over my face. I cried all the way home. How did it happen? How did our separation come about? Is it just because of the third person? I retraced our partnership painstakingly, searching for the origins of cracks in our love.

Certainly, I laughed a lot during our daily life; her negligence and stupid acts made me not know whether to laugh or cry. But, I committed a very serious mistake in our relationship. I got to know her after merely a month and began to date her within three months. Though I liked her a lot, perhaps it was because I constantly found myself remembering my ex-girlfriend and became immersed in the melancholia of the previous relationship. Yet as we got along with each other, she began to become an important part in my life in a way that I was unaware of.

I didn't realize how important she was to me until the day we broke up. I was so dependent on her and sucking greedily at the warmth she gave me. But I did not discover these facts; instead I was still wistful over the days with my ex-girlfriend and didn't give her much attention; this was one of the reasons that led to our separation.

PROGRESSION

I always said that it's the Matchmaker who brought us together. The Matchmaker is a deity responsible for romantic relationships in Taiwanese culture. I heard the Matchmaker in the Temple of City Gods in Wanwha brings the best hope for people. Having been single for almost four months, I was curious about it and thus invited a friend to go together for worship. Without adequate money to purchase the red silk (a symbol to connect couples), I could only pray in my mind: "To Matchmaker: I am a male-to-female transgendered person and I am sure you won't dismiss me just for this. I would like to request you bring a girlfriend to me. It is ok only if she is not bad-looking, suits me, and can accept transgender people while having an interest in gender/LBGTQ issues. Thank you very much." Thus, I achieved my goal in this small trip with half sincerity and a half attempt.

Two days later, I saw a message in the friend-making area of 5466, a bulletin board for lesbians:

"This is my first time requesting friends. I'm a poor student, but easy to get along with. Though I'm a bit busy, I still pay attention to sexuality/gender rights things sometimes. If you are interested in such issues also, maybe we can join any related activities together. It's kind of nice to have a partner like this."

I was excited to notice her mentioning "sexuality/gender rights things" and replied immediately. We got to know each other through discussions, sharing back and forth about LBGTQ issues, sex work issues, feminism issues, and our personal life experiences. But despite the joyful conversations, I still could not decide if or when I should tell her about my transgender identity.

Soon we had our first meeting in the Immigration Assembly Hall for a forum about sex/gender, media, and judicatory reform. In addition to us, her friend at school also attended the forum with her lover who was my first girlfriend. What's more, some of her classmates also had relations with me and my first girlfriend; the world was still small as before.

After the forum we went for dinner and discussed many subjects in a nearby restaurant. Talking face to face was in fact a little different from chatting on the Internet; from cyberspace to reality, we had to get to know each other again. With the progress of our dinner, the conversation became more active and the time disappeared more and more rapidly. "It's happy and sweet to talk to you on the Net, but only by meeting in person can the feelings we have be accurate and it went ok," she said afterwards.

The next day, we both participated in the anti-criminalization motorcade march for sex workers. The march's line was divided into different groups, and volunteers of Tawian's prostitute rights movement, the Collective of Sex Workers and Supporters (COSWAS) played special roles in special groups. I belonged to the sex worker-customer group, two persons per scooter. I played the role of a sex worker, while my customer (a familiar female friend, who was much taller and stronger than me) carried me on the scooter. My role forced me to be in an exposed costume, and I was very shy when encountering her as we just met the day before. I was also worried about my genitals being exposed due to my skimpy clothes, but luckily, it didn't happen. Some men in the crowd even flirted with me!

But something bad happened at the end of the march. I saw my ex-girlfriend acting in the street performance. Out of uneasiness, I intended to leave after watching her performance. Just at that moment, my ex-girlfriend delivered her passionate greetings. She called my name through the crowd, but I turned around spontaneously to avoid her eye contact. It was my ostrich policy, which helped me escape from the heart-breaking memories.

A few days later, I woke up in the middle of the night for no reason. A furious rage burned in me, and I could not fall back to sleep. I kept wondering how my ex-girlfriend could treat me in this way. She broke our promise, loved another person, and she dared to have the nerve to try and greet me. I knew that I didn't treat my ex very well. But at this moment, I lost control of my rage, and it burned more and more furiously. I failed to repress my emotions so I could no longer pretend as if nothing happened. The rage had been repressed for so long that it burst out all at once. I lost my last bit of self-control, and collapsed into this furious emotional flood. All I could do was wait. Wait for the flood to fade away in time.

Actually, ever since I identified myself as a transgender, I tried to find a way out for my repressed emotions. I experienced an extreme emotional breakdown after this march. Fortunately, because of my lovely chats with Internet girl, I gradually calmed myself down.

After the first encounter at the march, Internet girl and I met more and more frequently. We hung out every week just after we'd met on the Internet one month ago. "If she's the one who could accept my real identity, then I might come out at the right time; if she's not the one, then it's all right to be her friend," I thought to myself. One day, we went to the show "Super Drag Queen." Right before the show began, we were talking about transgenderism, a familiar topic between us. "We've discussed companionship in the class. What important things should be announced before two people get along with each other? Should one announce his or her school performance? Or, how about their transgender identity? Some of our classmates could not accept her lover to be a transgender," she said. Of course, this was before she knew my true identity.

With much anxiety, I asked, "Would you mind having a transgender lover?"

"I don't think so," she replied.

"Why not?"

"If I love someone, and can get along well with this person, gender is not a crucial concern."

"Oh . . . I see." I tried hard to keep myself from impulsively coming out.

I did it the next night instead. "I had a quarrel with my father," I complained to her.

"Mmm . . . is it about your homosexuality?" she asked.

"Not really. My relationship with my family is more complicated than you can imagine. I've been through lots of hardship, and it is more painful than you know, but I dare not tell you everything. Perhaps it's because I have no idea how to put it . . ."

"Okay . . ."

"Are you willing to listen?" All at once, I decided to uncover my true physical sex and transgender identity.

"Of course I am." Her reply encouraged me to tell her the truth.

"I've been keeping you from finding out who I am—in fact, I've hidden my real self from you, because I don't open up to others easily. But if you don't know my true self, it's hard for you to understand why I fight with my family."

"Okay, I am willing to listen."

"Thank you for trusting me so much." Thus, I trusted her from my deepest heart. "We've talked about several transgender issues, but I've never told you that transgender identity is part of me. That is why I fight with my family," I continued.

"Okay . . . Never mind. I don't mind your physical appearance. For me, it makes no difference if you're a boy or girl."

Hearing her reply, I suddenly saw the light. We talked a lot continuously, about my family, my school life, as if the time never ended. The following two days, we told each other everything about ourselves—her secrets, how she identified herself as a bisexual, my transgender body and its visibility, and so forth. And we became lovers.

She was slim and tender. She spoke with a soft voice, the sort of voice that you couldn't tell whether she was going to scream or shout. She gave me feelings of light kindness, sweetness, and intimacy. We understood each other very well, and often thought of the same thing in the same moment. We could tolerate each other's shortcomings ever since we fell in love. I kept reminding myself about the failures of my two previous affairs, and loved her with care. Hoping it would be a long-lasting relationship, we lived our lives with happiness.

Her parents didn't know much about her new affair. They only had a vague idea that she was dating a girl. Generally speaking, Taiwan's society is still conservative. Sexual diversity is visible to a certain extent, but it is not widely accepted. Family members usually attempt to "correct" LGBT children in their own ways, and for this reason, we keep our relationship a secret from her family.

As for me, although my family and relatives have gotten used to my transgender behaviors in these years, they never stop "correcting" me. Out of the attempt to make them better understand transgenderism, I invited my parents to Taipei to talk with my psychiatrist. Finally only my mom, grandma, and cousin came.

On the way to the hospital, my mom could not hide her curiosity. Thus, she asked my girlfriend, "Don't you worry that you can't have an ordinary marriage in the future? Okay, if you can accept a person like this, can your parents accept them?" With her greatest effort, my girlfriend explained why she decided to be supportive to me. Thanks to her, my mom was able to dispel some of her fears that I would have a lonely future.

Looking back on these three love affairs, I had three types of interaction with these girls: my first girlfriend was aggressive, agile, and with rich intimate experience. I was just like a dum-dum behind her back. In contrast, I behaved more aggressive than my second girlfriend. I usually made jokes about her. Her carefree lifestyle filled our life with laughter and humor. Now I am in my third relationship and I've got a richer love experience than before. To my girlfriend, I am a humorous and considerate lover. These girls I met influenced me a lot. They changed me, and made me grow up over these years, but of course they gave me more than that. Even if I didn't change a bit, I experienced different love styles with them, because every lover is unique, and I am unique, too.

My girlfriend and I get along well. Both of us are interested in gender and queer issues, and often attend conferences and activities together. In order to educate teachers and students about LGBT issues, we usually visit high schools and campuses to introduce the concepts of queer and transsexual by coming out. Besides, she also became a showgirl with the COSWAS, just like me. All of her attributes are in accord with what I prayed for to Matchmaker. Though we have not yet been together a year, it's my devout wish that we can be together for a long time. I really appreciate my lovers for everything they have given me. I cannot be what I am without your support.

15

Bodies May Lie but Hearts Never Do

Nickolas J. McDaniel

Dissecting my past from the position I now inhabit—the perspective of a successful, thirty-four-year-old graduate student who is white, heterosexual, male, and also a post-operative female-to-male transsexual (trans man or FTM)—I'm able to appreciate the changes I've made in my life and the great sacrifices needed in order to make these changes bear fruit.

Bodies may lie but the heart never does. Even though I was female-bodied for over three decades, I always identified as male. My heart always knew who I was; my gender identity was something I never questioned. My body told the world that I was female; it lied. Through masculinizing hormones, chest masculinization, and genital reconstruction surgery my body has become more congruent with my mind. The potential to be comfortable in my own skin is still such an abstract concept that my brain cannot quite fully grasp it. Inner peace is something I dreamed of but never quite dared believe I might actually achieve. It takes a very long time to overcome three decades of feeling wrong.

I am living proof that bodies *do* lie. Correcting my anatomical incongruence by transitioning has allowed me to deal with the past and start living my life at the age of thirty-two. Admittedly, it has been, and continues to be, the hardest and most rewarding thing I've ever done. I didn't invest all this time and money in myself because I was selfish; although still difficult to do so, I can finally grudgingly admit I'm worth the investment. Without these personal and financial sacrifices, I'd not be here today. I now live every moment as if it is my last.

Trans People In Love

I go to sleep each night with no regrets. As I see it, at thirty-four years of age I'm living on borrowed time. I wasn't supposed to live past thirty. It was only in the past year that I really began to live.

Although I began to notice girls in high school, I never dated. Unlike many trans men, I never identified as lesbian. I wasn't willing to give up who I was. No matter what lies my body told, my heart knew I was a heterosexual man, not a lesbian. Until I was nearly thirty years old I had no terms like "transsexual" to articulate how I felt. Being seen by a potential girlfriend as female was a risk I couldn't take. Before 2005, I never dated; I shut my sexuality off and isolated myself.

There is a tendency among normatively-gendered people who have never experienced incongruence between their mental and physical gender to confuse gender identity, sex, and sexual orientation. Although all three share points of commonality, they are separate things. Considering how little dialogue actually occurs in contemporary, mainstream media and education regarding these topics, this confusion is not surprising. Many people use "gender" and "sex" interchangeably, erroneously thinking that gender is a more politically correct or socially polite term than sex. In addition, many believe that gender identity and sexual orientation are the same. They aren't.

How can we as a society begin to talk about something when the basic definitions are unknown or diversely defined by the majority of people? How can we begin to question gender when many people don't understand what it is and share a common definition? In order to explain my sexual personal growth as it relates to my transness, I pause here to establish a common ground. Here's the simple breakdown of sex, gender, and sexual orientation as I understand and will be using these terms.

Sex is one's biological, physical anatomy. It's how things look "down there." It's the possession of male or female genitalia (external and internal), or in the case of people who are intersexed, a mix and match of the two. It can also be used to refer to intercourse or other intimate sexual acts, but I won't be using it in that context. Gender identity is an individual's own psychological sense of being masculine, feminine, or androgynous regardless of their birth genitalia or sex. It is possible to be a masculine woman or feminine male. Gender identity influences what one wears and the gender role someone takes. Sexual orientation is determined by the gender, sex, or sexes (in the case of bisexuals) of the people an individual is attracted to romantically.

The three terms defined above are all interdependent and share some overlap. This commonality, and the way they are or aren't taught and spoken of, is the reason for the misconception that sex, sexual orientation, and gender identity are the same. Now that I've established a common ground, I can explain how I, a trans man, have grown romantically.

I've learned one of the sweetest fruits life has to offer is love. Love found me when I was looking so hard for it I had no idea I already had it. In April 2005 I got an e-mail from a woman I'd met in a transsexual support group in Monterey, California. Her name was Sonia. We'd been hanging out a lot since she first entered the group in January 2005. A twenty-four year-old undergraduate student at California State University–Monterey Bay (CSUMB), she slowly but surely got me to come out of my room. This was impressive. Even though I was a full-time third-year undergraduate student living at Oakes College on the University of California–Santa Cruz campus (UCSC), I still kept to myself. I was a loner and geek most likely to hold up a wall if someone was persistent enough to get me to go. That was a big if. My spare time was spent hiding in my room behind a personal computer, finishing assignments early so I could edit other people's papers for fun. Socializing was a lesson so intimidating I'd not yet mastered it.

Others had tried to get me out before with no success. Sonia succeeded where they'd failed. We had a deep connection on several levels that neither of us understood. I allowed her to hug me hello and goodbye whereas with other people I still freaked out and ran away. As a male survivor of sexual abuse, the only touch I'd ever received had hurt me deeply. Fight as I might, Sonia was slowly teaching me to crave healthy human touch even though I still feared it.

I thought we were just good friends; She thought we were dating. After we went to see *The Aviator* at the Northridge Cinema in my hometown of Salinas, California and spent an afternoon on the UCSC campus, she realized just how clueless I really was.

Before that time, I'd always gone to the movies with my brother. We had our little movie-going ritual. I'd follow him to whatever seats he'd picked. He'd sit down. I'd sit one seat over. We'd put our jackets in the empty seat in the middle, sprawl, and watch the movie. I had no reason to believe going to the movies with Sonia would be any different. I learned the hard way how it's supposed to be when you go with a girl.

I expressed interest in seeing *The Aviator*. She said she hadn't seen it (though she had seen it several months prior to its theatrical release). We went. She sat down. I sat one seat over and put my jacket in the unoccupied middle one, sprawled, and then watched the movie. Sonia was livid. I had no idea. I just thought the special effects in the flight scenes lacked realism. In response, Sonia sent me the following e-mail on Friday, March 25, 2005:

> You've confused me! In a good way though. Part of me thinks it's a crush, another part thinks it's because we relate in a way that I haven't been able to with anyone else. I wanted to bring this up because it's been occupying my mind an awful lot lately. Regardless I am very glad that we are friends and I hope that no matter what, we will always be friends.

My reaction? Shock. I scanned the e-mail. I was sure I'd misread it. There had to have been a "not" in front of "a crush." If so, look as I might, I was unable to find it. For over three decades I'd always been morbidly obese, horrifically abused, and told how wrong I was. Even though I'd lost almost two hundred pounds, my self-esteem was still poor. The thought of someone—much less an extremely cute and intelligent someone like Sonia—with a crush on an awkward, uncoordinated, painfully shy me was something I'd never prepared for. Confused, scared, and panicked, I shut my computer down.

I woke up with an extremely bad bout of bronchitis the next morning. That bought me time to think. I sent her an e-mail telling her I was sick but I'd get back to her on that. I literally turned off my computer and didn't touch it much for the two weeks I was sick. This fact alone—that I shut off and avoided my computer for two weeks—demonstrates just how ill-prepared I was. I'm seldom far from my computer. I used every excuse I could to postpone replying as I thought over the following two weeks. Think I did.

As mom had pointed out, Sonia was cute and we did get along really well. My brother also had a good point: what did I have to lose? I couldn't deny I was attracted to her. I'm embarrassed to admit in my confusion and panic over those two weeks, my befuddled, feverish brain was also a bit hypocritical; the fact that she, herself, was a male-to-female transsexual (trans woman or MTF) had me questioning my sexual orientation. Did this mean I was a trannie chaser? Had I violated the sanctity of the group to use it to pick up on attendees? Did anyone in it know? However, that dilemma lasted about an hour or two; Sonia was very much a girl and my motivation for attending the group was innocent and appropriate. The main mental obstacle I had to overcome was being torn between my fears of trusting or maybe even loving someone and the profound loneliness I'd not previously realized. I had never needed anyone before. The thought of letting Sonia in terrified me, but in the end, the thought of not letting her in terrified me more.

Once I'd recovered from bronchitis and my insecurities, I finally agreed to go to Emo Tendencies. It was Sonia's Friday night radio slot on the CSUMB student radio station from 10 p.m. till midnight. She played emo and punk music there to fulfill a class requirement after she got off work. I agreed to meet her at her apartment and ride to the on-campus station.

I was totally scared! I comforted myself with a speech I had all planned out. Although so nervous I felt like I was going to throw up, I would sound really slick! I must've gone over it twenty times on the thirty-minute drive between my house in Salinas and her apartment in Marina, California. By the time I walked up the stairs to her place I had it all worked out. The plan was to sound suave and cool. Take my time. Wait for just the right moment, recite my speech looking cool and not too interested, and then . . . well, I hadn't gotten that far in my planning because I didn't rightly know what to do. Like any pubescent boy I had some good ideas what I *wanted* to do but not how to get there.

Throughout her show and afterwards while hanging out in her apartment, I was painfully aware of the ticking clock. It was after midnight. I was still waiting for just the right moment to happen but it never seemed to. The more time that passed, the louder the clock seemed to tick. The louder it got, the more I began to sweat. I was frantic. I knew if I didn't do something soon, I'd chicken out and be alone for the rest of my life. The thought of returning not just tonight but every night to my empty room with only my computer for company—it was more than I could bear. Sonia's e-mails had opened doors to possibilities that, once opened, could never be closed again.

Around 1 a.m., I could stand it no longer. I had to make a move. I hoarsely croaked out the first line of my speech. Even though it never had before, my voice wavered and cracked (or at least to my ears it did) but the first couple of words of my speech sounded beautiful! Verbal poetry! My confidence soared until . . . her blue eyes looked at me steamily from under her eyelids. I looked at her. I lost my thoughts in those sparkling pools of hers. "Oh. My. God." I thought. "She's looking at me!" In that moment Sonia was the most beautiful woman I had ever seen.

Suddenly I couldn't remember what planet I was on or how to speak, much less the cool speech I had all planned out. What the hell was I going to say? She was sitting there, waiting in so much dead air. This was supposed to be memorable, yet here I sat, trapped before I started by fear. Beads of sweat popped out on my forehead, each pore a huge reservoir full of jiggling, salty panic. My tongue was like a stick of dead beef jerky. No matter how hard I tried to make it work, it just lay there pasted to the roof of my mouth, thick and stupid like me. My brain frantically screamed, "She's waiting!!! Say something, stupid! Anything! You're going to blow it!"

With hands that weren't quite steady, I picked up the book sitting by me on her bed. Ironically, I think it was her copy of the fourth edition of the *Diagnostic and Statistical Manual of Mental Disorders*. To this day, I honestly have no clue if it was right side up or upside down. Either way it doesn't matter. It had the desired effect. I was so used to spending my life hiding behind a book or laptop that it really helped to have something to hide behind. My tongue dislodged from the roof of my mouth with an audible "riiiiip!" as the dried saliva released it. I finally managed to say, "So I thought, uhm . . . what the hell." My brain screamed, "Stupid! Stupid! Stupid! That was NOT anywhere in the speech!"

It actually took me all weekend to figure out if she did get my message. My original speech might never have gotten airtime, but the mission was accomplished. She heard me loud and clear. I finally had my very first girlfriend—my very first love. With her e-mail, male puberty began for me. My range of emotions broadened. My heart opened wide. Both of us knew and understood through personal experience that bodies lie but the heart never does. Before Sonia's e-mail I had known only various depths and degrees of depression; now there was a huge spectrum of emotions I'd never known existed. As a writer, it was frustrating to have a feeling for the first time in my life but be at a loss for words to describe it beyond good, hurt, or bad.

Overnight my libido went from nothing to a state of nearly constant arousal, just like that of a pubescent boy. I began to grow as a human being and as a man socially and mentally—the growth I'd been denied prior to transition. This was hard, confusing, and wonderful all at the same time.

Sonia and I dated until September 2005. With her I experienced my first kiss, my first trip outside of California, my first new car, my first taste of beer, my first stage of phalloplasty, the first time someone told me, "I love you" and meant it. It was intense, passionate, loving, confusing, stressful, terrifying and, at times, a psychotic feeling. I'd not exchange those months for anything—it was a priceless time I'll always remember fondly. I used to feel like the king of the world when she'd call me "sweetie" or "Prince of Princes."

In the end, we were just too close, the issues we struggled with too similar. We each had a lot of growing up to do in order to be ready for as serious a relationship as we were in. The intense pain was such that I'd never experienced before. I was not prepared for it to end; I still loved her deeply. We remained close, just not romantically. To this day I feel like Sonia is closer to me than anyone in this world in many ways; I imagine she would say the same. My love for her has deepened and grown over time, as have I.

When we broke up I was interning for academic credit at a nonprofit organization in Santa Cruz called Triangle Speakers. They wanted me to go to the local Santa Cruz Trans Support meeting on October fourth. My objective? Do outreach, speak from my heart to those present about how it felt to speak about the experience of being transsexual and try to encourage people to volunteer and be trained speakers. Little did I know I'd recruit more than a good speaker that night.

Three-fourths of my way through my recruitment speech, three women walked in late. Damn! I had to start my spiel over again. Honestly, I didn't mind so much. I was inspired. Two of these girls caught my eye. They were cute! I didn't know how to do it, but I knew I wanted their e-mail addresses. It was something I'd never done before. Though I needed to be up early the next day, I ended up staying late and tagging along with the group to the Saturn Cafe. Finally I decided to resolve myself to failure. It was getting late and I was no closer to my goal than I'd been four hours earlier. As I got up to leave, one woman passed a slip of paper over the table, the second under the table. I drove home a very happy man. I had no idea if either was actually interested in me as just a friend or something more.

Sonia ended up being the one who told me one of those girls, Jacqui, was interested in me. They knew each other casually through a trans community on an online blog called Live Journal. So after a few nights of exchanging long instant message conversations on the computer, I asked Jacqui out.

Jacqui became my second girlfriend. She also became good friends with Sonia. Yes, they bonded over me and gleefully enjoy torturing me mercilessly as they compare notes. Jacqui and I have now been together for over a year. I've watched her become an eloquent speaker. She has also accompanied me to Nashville for stages two and three of my phalloplasty. In June 2006, I was there for her in Thailand as she recovered from her own surgery. Jacqui has listened to me speak about my transition at countless speaking engagements, watched me graduate from the University of California–Santa Cruz and begin my pursuit of certification as a sex therapist and gender specialist. Each moment, no matter how momentous or mundane, is always special when I'm able to share it with her. It definitely feels different than my relationship with Sonia, but no less special, memorable, or wonderful. Jacqui continues the hard work Sonia started: to teach me how to love.

Through knowing and loving these two wonderful women, I've grown as a man and a human being. Through the struggles they have, I've become aware of issues facing MTFs. They have also made me aware of the institutionalized discrimination women live with each and every day. Because I never identified nor tried to live as female, I was previously unaware of it. They impress on me the fact that I never was a girl. As I come to discover and define what being a man means to me, these women help me find my heart and myself. They each patiently support me as I recover from issues of the past such as abuse and gender dysphoria. They've become my role models and I love them both for that. Most importantly love has reiterated one lesson I learned long ago as a child in regards to being transsexual: bodies may lie but ultimately the heart never does.

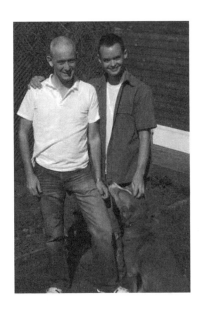

Nick Laird (right) with his partner, Mark and their dog, Floyd.

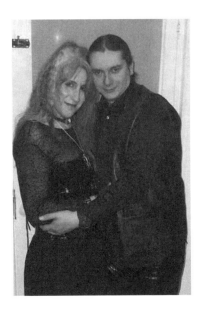

Debra Hastings (left) and her partner, David.

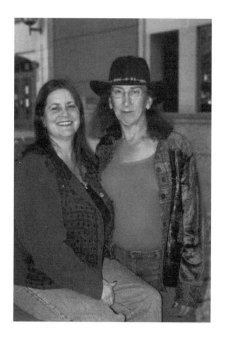

Gypsey Teague (right) with her wife, Marla.

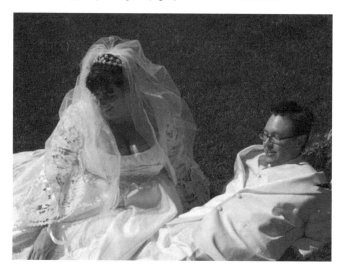

Jacob Anderson-Minshall (right) with his wife, Diane, on their wedding day. Photo by Kina Williams

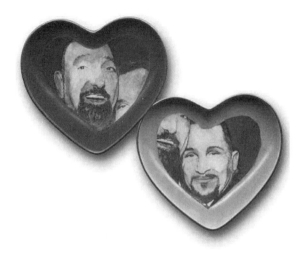

Jordy Jones (below right), and his partner, Alan (the heart-shaped trays were a gift from Alan to Jordy).

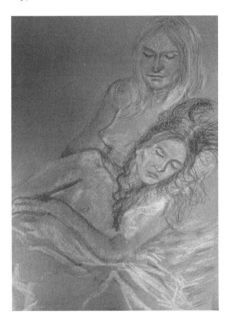

Kayla Karstens (left) and her partner, Laura. Drawing by Gabrielle Le Roux.

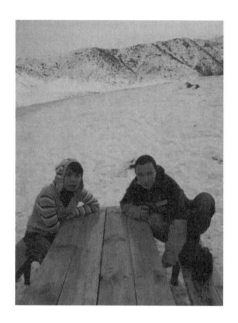

Orsekov Dan (right) and his partner, Regina.

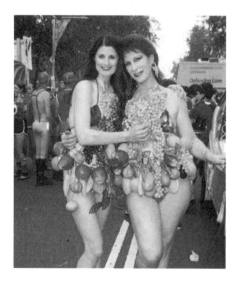

Tracie O'Keefe (right) and her partner, Katrina Fox, at the Sydney Gay and Lesbian Mardi Gras Parade, 2007.

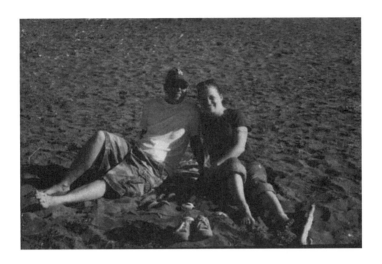

Zayne Jones (left) and his partner, Tami.

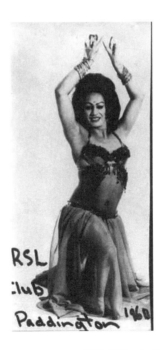

Carmen at the Paddington RSL Club, Sydney in 1960.

16

Satan and Lady Babalon: Polyamory Again at 64

Rusty Mae Moore, PhD

I started this little memoir in August 2006, when I was a sixty-four-year-old post-op woman of transsexual experience. I have been in a committed relationship with another woman of transsexual experience for the past fifteen years. We have described our relationship since early on as "one of the great love stories for the ages."

We were both pre-op when we met, although I was not yet fully out, while Chelsea, my partner, had been out and a queer activist for many years. She was Goth, and a minor celebrity in the hip community of Greenwich Village. I was a college professor, parent of three, living on suburban Long Island. She was thirty-one, and I was forty-nine.

When I saw her it was love at first sight. She walked into the bedroom where I was with my then lover Kelly, and her ex-lover, wearing black motorcycle boots, black jeans, a black silk camisole, a black leather jacket with the words "Take a Transsexual to Lunch" painted on the back, and a black Stetson with a flat brim. She was smoking a long, thin cheroot, and wearing a loaded pack frame that contained her life possessions. She was 6'4" and slim as a rail.

With one look I left Kelly's side on the bed and took several steps toward her before I realized what I was doing. Without a word passing between us I understood that we were kindred spirits. I think it was the backpack that did it.

Our relationship developed in the shared experiences of the prostitution-centered drag clubs of New York, the transition-oriented "Survivors of Transsexuality Anonymous" twelve-step group at the New York City Lesbian, Gay, Bisexual, and Transgender Community Center, and the long nights we shared making love in my suburban apartment. We always thought of ourselves as lesbians.

Chelsea was between homes at the time, and soon moved in with me. As a lesbian couple we developed an image in the drag subculture at Sally's II in Times Square, the same culture which was documented in the film *Paris Is Burning*. Open lesbian trans couples were the exception rather than the rule among the "working" she-males in those days. We would dance erotically in the ballroom of the Carter Hotel, while the Johns and the other girls watched and commented.

In 1994 we moved to Park Slope, Brooklyn, where I had purchased a small townhouse. This place soon became known as "Transy House," a center of political action and trans cultural expression, as well as a home for homeless trans women who came to live with us.

Chelsea and I had a loose three-way relationship with Kelly for a time, and then a more serious relationship with another person, Julia. We were lovers for only about three years, but the three of us lived in the same communal space at Transy House as close friends for most of the past twelve years.

Chelsea and I had sex-change surgery in Brussels in the summer of 1995, lying side by side in the hospital and in the Derby Hotel as we convalesced. When we returned to Brooklyn our love relationship went through a crisis. We were both still bisexual, but she became more oriented toward women, and I became more oriented toward men than we had been previously. I told Chelsea that I wanted to develop relationships with men as we lay in bed one evening. She did not want this, asking why I had let her have a sex change if I wanted a man. She sprang from the bed, grasped a box cutter lying on her dresser, and slashed her wrist with a sickening, whistling sound, saying that she did not want to live if I wanted to throw her over for a man, especially a "transfan" type of man.

I went into a monumental rage that she would do this to me, but I took her to the hospital emergency room for seventeen stitches. When I cooled down and examined my feelings I came to the realization that she meant more to me in the deep relationship that we had than did some unknown man in the mists of the future. I realized that no relationship goes forward without some loving discipline and sacrifice. We stayed together, and our closeness developed apace. Over the next twelve years we were the co-mothers of Transy House, participated in trans-activism, traveled in Latin America and Europe, played and performed music together, read a lot of books together, and studied hermetic philosophy in Amsterdam. Our families and our work colleagues came to see us as a couple. Many people forgot which one was Chelsea and which one was Rusty.

In 2003 Chelsea changed for a time into Chet, a male-like person, and I faced the issues experienced by lesbians who have their partner "go FTM." This period did not last, although after I adjusted to it, I liked it.

Our relationship was "open." Chelsea had periodic relationships with other women, and I would once in a while have a quickie with a man I had picked up in an S&M club. I knew that Chelsea felt hurt when I periodically came in late, or if she saw the marks of whips or ropes on my body. Chelsea was a jealous lover, and to appease her I dropped some of the long-standing close relationships I had had with both women and men friends. We had a close intellectual bond. Chelsea turned me on to science fiction, to paganism, and to jazz. I turned her on to international travel, and gave her a financial security that she had never had before.

In the spring of 2006 our plans were focused on emigrating to the Netherlands after my retirement from teaching in Spring 2007. Chelsea was the big impetus for this. We had spent a July and a January in the past year in the Netherlands and thought we knew what the country had to offer. We were taking several hours of Dutch lessons each week, and we were in the slow processes of rearranging our affairs in the U.S. Chelsea and I were sharing the experience of being grandparents to Caleb, my daughter Amanda's first child. Chelsea had long since been integrated into the flow of family affairs with my three children who also lived in Brooklyn. I had accepted a steady monogamy with Chelsea, and felt a constant deepening in our relationship as we shared our lives together. I had no doubt by this time that my relationship with Chelsea was the closest of the three extended marriages, all with women, that I have had in my life. It was amazing to me that the sex was still hot between us.

Chelsea had been undergoing a spiritual transition in recent years. She had moved away from Christianity and turned back strongly toward pagan roots. Our periods in the Netherlands involved deeper studies at the Rittman Library of Hermetic Philosophy in Amsterdam, and at the Amsterdam Theosophical Society. I read many of the works that she suggested.

Back in the U.S., Chelsea was inducted as a Priestess of Isis in Winter 2006, and by the Spring of 2006 was elevated as a Priestess of Cybele at the Maetreum of Cybele in the Catskill Mountains of New York. She took her elevation as a Cybelline priestess seriously. She explained to me that she would be spending a considerable amount of time at the "spiritual community" in the Catskill Mountains, and would be apart from me quite often if I did not go there with her. I accepted this as a not unwelcome chance to be alone, and was not disquieted by being apart from her periodically.

All of the above is background for the profound change that came to our relationship in June 2006. These changes are still being worked out, my emotions are still raw and uncertain, and the future cannot be foretold. The paragraphs below are merely a status report on the current direction of our relationship.

In early June I arrived at the Maetreum of Cybele to spend the weekend with Chelsea, and to take her back to Brooklyn for a week or so. When I arrived I was shocked that Chelsea had effectively moved in with Katrina, a young trans woman who had recently come to live at the Maetreum. Kat and Chelsea were referring to each other as "wife," and were pledging to be with each other for the rest of their lives. Chelsea would stay with me at night until I went to sleep, perhaps making love with me, but then would go off to spend the night with Kat.

I tried to have self-discipline so that I could handle these changes with equanimity. I had often had flashes of jealousy when a series of people over the years made passes at Chelsea, but I had always felt that these were just dalliances for her, and that in the end she would come back to me. Kat was different. She was young, less than half my age, beautiful, and highly intelligent. Beyond that, she had an allure for Chelsea that I could not match in any way. She was Goth; she was dark; she is a daughter of Kali; she is a vampire; she drinks the blood of Chelsea, and Chelsea drinks the blood of Kat.

I felt powerless, betrayed, and abandoned. I was old, flabby, wrinkling, and failing mentally. I felt as if Chelsea had taken up with the new love of her life before I had completely left the scene. Chelsea used the same words of endearment with Kat that she had been using with me for a long time. Instead of feeling as if I were the center of

Chelsea's universe as I always had, I suddenly felt like a used-up old shoe.

Chelsea did assure me that she would be glad to have me join the two of them if I wished. I could not do this, as I barely knew Kat, and got no signal from her that she did anything more than tolerate me with a kind of unconcern originating in her certainty that Chelsea was ultimately hers. Chelsea assured me that she still loved me, and that things would not change. I told her that everything had changed, and that we were now operating under a new paradigm.

I returned to Brooklyn without Chelsea and with a sense of angry, hurt, agitation. I went to the Alt.com S&M site and renewed my profile. To my surprise, quite a few men seemed to be very interested in meeting me in spite of my age and status as a woman of transsexual experience. With trepidation I met a young man of thirty, and we ended up having a delightful erotic experience. I visited overnight in the Pocono Mountains at the home of an acquaintance and had a lovely time, which he also seemed to enjoy. I went out with some other men. My sense of personal attractiveness was renewed. I finally gained confidence in my relationships with men, and I did not feel old and used up anymore.

Upon reflection I realized that I felt really bleak. One-night stands are nothing compared to a deeper, passionate love with a soulmate. The thought of not having time with Chelsea left me feeling as if I faced a void. I was desperate to have a continuing closeness with her even if "my minutes were cut," as they say in basketball.

Chelsea had initiated me as "The Whore of Babalon" in a ceremony inspired by Aleister Crowley's Order of the Temple of the East in Amsterdam in January 2006 ("Babalon" is the Crowley spelling, as opposed to "Babylon"). I felt joy and peace in seeing myself as her avatar; it suited me in a way that nothing else ever had. In the process of my dalliances with men on my rebound from Chelsea and Kat, I lived out my role as the "Lady Babalon." I concentrated on opening without reserve to any partner I was with, trying to get my very soul in touch with theirs, and to heal them if I could.

My friends and family in Brooklyn were outraged that Chelsea would take up with a new partner without even mentioning the possibility to me beforehand. My three children were hostile to Kat and mad at Chelsea.

I continued to commute to the Catskills on the weekends through-out the summer. In mid-July we all went to the National Organization for Women (NOW) conference in nearby Albany. There we allied with the sex workers of the Desiree Alliance who were trying to get the NOW people to adopt a sex-worker positive program. By this time I was relating more easily with Chelsea and Kat, but the two of them were mostly entwined together. At one point, one of the women invited Chelsea and "her partner" (i.e., Kat) to come to an after-hours party. This invitation was like a knife through my heart after so long as Chelsea's only partner. To the outside world I kept a stiff upper lip, but sunk to the depths of enlisting sympathy for my plight from old friends.

Later, as Chelsea and I lay together before she went to Kat's bed I mentioned to her how I felt when Kat was acknowledged as her part-ner, and then I broke into abandoned sobs. I wailed harder than I ever had in my life. Chelsea said that she too had felt badly about the situa-tion.

The next day, on the day of my return to Brooklyn, I took Chelsea's invitation to share the bed in Kat's room. I felt desperate. I felt that I had to accept a polyamorous relationship because I would otherwise lose Chelsea completely. In some ways I felt as if Chelsea had grown far beyond me. As the three of us lay there, Chelsea initiated a water ceremony which made the three of us water-sisters, following Hein-lein's *Stranger in a Strange Land*. It was a nice day laying with the two of them. I asked humbly with tears in my eyes if Chelsea could be with me sometimes.

Over July and August the three of us spent a good deal of time to-gether. We moved together into a two-room suite at the Maetreum, and bought a huge king-sized memory foam mattress so that we could all sleep comfortably together. Kat and I had a cordial relationship, and I found that she had many ways of thinking and being that were similar to mine. I more or less adopted the advice of Jamie, an old friend and spiritual mentor, that I was "very lucky to have two beautiful wives."

I felt terrible for Kat from the standpoint of how the authorities had torn her young daughter from her, stripped her of parental rights for the crime of being transsexual in Alabama, and put the child up for adoption. My heart went out to Kat when I thought of how they had put her into a solitary cell for three months, allowing her one hour of light out of each twenty-four, and then on the ninety-first day had released her with no charges. I felt that Kat needed love so much, and that she wanted so much to come back from the post-traumatic stress disorder which possessed her. I wanted to help her with a sense of loving, more parental than amorous.

On one level I felt that my love for Chelsea was such that I wanted to not get in the way of her love of Kat. Both of them needed the relationship. I wanted to encourage them in a way that almost seemed perverse to me. On another level I thought of Kat as a good way for Chelsea to assure her future as I entered old age and death. In truth, I also appreciated the greater freedom I had been given to explore my bisexuality instead of repressing it.

The sexual relationship between Chelsea and me leaped upward at the same time that I was fighting through my waves of feelings of abandonment and jealousy. Chelsea and I had always had a good sexual relationship, but she was almost always the initiator. In my new spirit I cherished Chelsea in a way I previously had not. With me, Chelsea had always fallen into a more butch, aggressor role. With Kat, Chelsea seemed to feel more feminine. She dressed in a more feminine manner and seemed to be willing to take a less dominant sexual role. I suddenly, perhaps released by my sense of being an avatar of the Whore of Babalon, was able to adopt and enjoy a more aggressive role with her. Our lovemaking went to new heights and our spirituality was greatly enhanced. At the end of August 2006 I had reached the point of writing the following:

> As of this writing I feel happier in my relationship with Chelsea, and more comfortable in my relationship with Kat. She has even said that she loves me, although I have not yet reciprocated. We have kissed once or twice, and I have caressed her a bit. Chelsea still sleeps between us, however. I am intrigued by being once again in a polyamorous relationship. I cannot imagine where it may be going, but indications are that the present direction is positive. I am even thinking of adopting a "Goth grandmother in combat boots" look. Chelsea and Kat sometimes describe us as "the professor and her two science experiments."

Over the next several months Kat retreated into the space of two rooms which she shared with Chelsea and me in the pagan spiritual communal home in the Catskill Mountains north of New York City where we lived. Chelsea gradually came to feel restricted within this lifestyle, and began to spend most of her time accompanying me at our house in Brooklyn when I was not at the Catskill Mountain home. Kat and I developed a stronger bond of friendship during this period, and our triple relationship became more comfortable for me.

Gina came on the scene in mid-November, another tall, slim trans woman in her mid-thirties who dressed in black. Chelsea and Gina developed a love relationship which included me in its sexual aspects, and I enjoyed Gina's friendship. Kat was very friendly toward Gina at first, but soon began to feel betrayed that Chelsea was spending so much time with Gina outside the small personal space in which Kat felt comfortable. By January 2007 Chelsea and Gina were announcing that they were in love, and intended to be together as they went through life. I definitely had twinges of jealousy about Gina, although much weaker than I had experienced with Kat. Chelsea constantly assured me that I was one of her primary relationships, and Gina seemed to be very pleased when I joined them. Kat, on the other hand, seemed to feel excluded by Chelsea and Gina, and expressed dissatisfaction that Chelsea would not talk honestly with her about the new relationship.

I felt sorry that Kat felt betrayed and excluded. I tried to reach out to her and reassure her. Chelsea had created the concept of the three of us being in a "nest" which I went along with, but was skeptical about. Now I had become the one trying to hold the nest together, adding Gina as a fourth, rather than replacing Kat with Gina. This is where we stand today, in mid-February, 2007. I cannot say that I have a passionate love with either Kat or Gina, but I am fond of them, and feel friendship with them. Perhaps we will fall in love, or maybe into the pattern of polyamorous relationships, which include primary and secondary relationships. It continues to be hard to widen my emotional space from embracing a couple relationship to a quadruple relationship, even while my conscious intellect embraces the idea, and expresses the view that love relationships are infinitely expandable. I learned years ago that love is an endless source of energy, not a fixed source that must be doled out in little chunks. Love between two people does not need to detract from each of them loving other people. We are all trying to learn this and make it the guiding knowledge of our lives.

Perhaps Chelsea and I can still say that ours is one of the great love stories of the ages. She says that our nest is a very spiritual thing. I ask her what it means that I am Lady Babalon. She says, "The Whore of Babylon is the bride of Satan, and I am . . . ?" I always feel good when she says this.

17

The Adventures of a Trans Man in Love, Sex, and Spirituality

Joseph J. Nutini

We met on many occasions before actually getting together. The first time was six years ago in a McDonald's where she used to work. I was dating her ex and had just moved to Tucson from Chicago. Our eyes met with an intensity that I was too quick to deny. I wasn't ready for what she had to offer and so we parted ways.

Over the next couple of years we met in passing at various events held by the local lesbians, gays, bisexuals, and transgender (LGBT) group. Our eyes would meet as we stood close by. I thought that she'd never go for me. After all, at that time she was the hottest trannyboi in Tucson and was going by the name David. I was just a newbie. No one knew me or knew that I too was trans. He was in the newspapers and I was just a student at the university studying women's studies. David and I never spoke or worked on anything together. Only occasionally our eyes would meet and mine would lower. In the fall of 2002 all that changed.

It was that semester that I first became close friends with David's partner, Anita (who later transitioned to male as well). She took to me instantly. We became quick friends and she helped me through many milestones of transitioning including coming out and dealing with cutting issues because of body hatred. Needless to say it was a rough time.

As the school year progressed I started to hang out with Anita more and more. As a result I also saw more of David. What was strange about this time was that David and I never had a chance to interact

Trans People In Love

alone. It was like fate did not want us to really talk and bond with one another then. David and Anita invited me over to their home many times, helped me win a drag pageant and just served as my friends. They helped me come to terms with being transgender. It was much needed but still quite hard.

When we graduated, some strange things began to happen. Anita began to tell me that David was controlling her and that she wanted to come live with me. I helped her with that. Then she started dating David again and telling me that she loved me as well. I had heard of and practiced polyamory in the past and wondered if that was what she was referring to. It was, but what resulted was polyamory gone badly.

Anita, who at this time started going by the name Alan (and by masculine pronouns), began playing a series of mind games with us. He basically told David that I wanted to hurt him physically and told me that David hated me. I believed it and so did he. Then later Alan came clean to both of us and told us that he said that because he believed that if David and I were intimate we would fall in love with each other.

When I heard the last statement I was shocked. David was a guy. Granted he was very feminine but still identified as male. I, on the other hand, was very masculine in comparison and had never fallen for a man. The fact that Alan lied didn't bother me though. Since he told the truth he also told me of his feelings for the both of us and how he wanted the three of us to go on a date with each other. I figured, "What the hell?" The worse that could happen is that it wouldn't work out.

So, I planned a date of pizza and video games. It had been a while since I had seen David and I remember being very nervous. As soon as we got to the place my nervousness seemed to go away. We were actually having fun! I was actually being treated like a man! We went back to my place with the intentions of having sex but it didn't happen that night.

This date sparked three of the most passionate months I have ever had in my life. It was filled with dates, loving, passionate sex, and fun. At the same time, Alan still had not let David and I be alone. It was hard to be passionate alone with Alan, with Alan and David at the same time, but never with David alone. I grew weary and something told me that there was a game being played in this relationship. I knew that polyamory never seemed to work without near-total honesty. While I loved Alan, I didn't trust him for some reason.

One day after a long fight with Alan I was supposed to go to put up stock at my father's store. Instead, I drove down to David's apartment and approached the front door. I remember my heart pounding deep inside my chest as my finger pushed the buzzer to let him know someone was there. I no longer thought David was better than me. The issue was I didn't know what to think. While I had a deep, loving connection to this person I also realized that Alan was preventing us from becoming close. My finger let go and I waited in anticipation for David to answer.

"Hello?" he said questioningly.

"Hey dude, it's Joe. I need to talk to you. Can I come up?" I asked quickly.

"Uh . . . yeah," he said with a great deal of uncertainty.

The elevator ride up to the floor where the apartment was seemed to take an eternity. He was there waiting for me as the elevator doors opened. I looked at him and tears formed in my eyes. He put his arm around me and guided me to his apartment. I realized that I was so very tired.

As soon as we entered the lounge I sat down on his couch and began pouring my soul out to him. First, I spoke about being a trans man and being scared to transition. Then I cried over the horrible periods, bleeding, and cramps I had since I was sixteen. After that we began talking about Alan and learning that he had been playing games with us the whole time. We weren't sure what to do so we held hands lightly for awhile and then made a plan that involved me talking to Alan.

The rest of the summer was difficult. David was evicted from his apartment and we were all living in the same place. Alan became very distant after we learned of his deception and would not listen to us say we loved him. Eventually he left for home and did not return for almost three years. He later told me that he could not handle it. He just wasn't ready. I didn't blame him because I had been there myself. However, I still wonder what kind of passionate love the three of us could have had and sometimes I feel some lingering hurt.

Now, what was funny about the interaction between David and I was that we had never admitted our love for one another. I think part of it was that I was not sure I was ready to be in a relationship with "another man." David knew he was ready but just didn't know how to tell me. It was like the tables were turned. He was now the one who was scared to talk to me. We lived together as friends for a while.

About four months after graduation I had a job interview in Las Vegas for a very large corporation. I invited David to go with me. We went to Vegas on a wonderful trip in a cool rental car and we stayed in cheap yet awesome hotels. During that time we played an interesting little game. We would sleep in the bed together but wouldn't have sex. We had yet to have sex together alone.

Well, on the way back during our trip we stopped in beautiful Sedona, Arizona. It was dark and we could not find a hotel. I needed to stop driving to stretch so I pulled over near the forest. It was pitch black except for the bright starts. David came over to the side of the car where I was standing and suddenly put his arm around my shoulder. I felt a chill go down my spine and all I could do was put my arms around his waist.

"I'm scared out here in the dark," he said in all seriousness.

I touched his face lightly and smiled, "What? Don't be silly. I will protect you." Then I leaned forward, pushed his body against the car and kissed him with all the passion that I could muster. That kiss seemed to last for an eternity and it was the sweetest kiss I have ever had in my life. Of course, being the tough guy that I was back then, I didn't tell him that. I just smiled, pulled open the car door and told him to get in. That same night we finally found a hotel in Sedona. It was an absolutely beautiful place. I didn't let David come in with me because I wanted to get one bed. I didn't want him to know my plans.

See, the reality was that I had wanted to be alone with him for quite some time. During one of our threesomes we were all cuddling and I was rubbing his head (he was bald for a short period) making jokes. Inside, all I could think about was how I was starting to love this person and how sexy he was. It scared me. I liked it. Well, he entered our room first and I followed behind him. When he saw one bed he turned to me and gave me the sweetest, most submissive look I had ever seen in my life. It reminded me of something he had said to me.

"I've always wanted a daddy," he had said.

I took him gently in my arms at first, with caution. See, both of us had been abused pretty badly in our lives. Much of the abuse came from our past romantic relationship. I knew this so I didn't want to hurt him at all. We kissed and touched, softly at first, just exploring. Still, I had a great deal of hesitation.

Suddenly he said, "Daddy will you please fuck me?"

I didn't need to be asked twice. That night I fucked him while making love at the same time. With him a passion and a new hope was ignited in me like never before. I felt suddenly like I had met a girl for my boy parts and a boy for my girl parts. See, while I identify as mostly male I know there is a girl part to my spirit. That night David touched all of me. That night I knew I had found a taste of true love.

I want to jump ahead a bit and tell you about the past year of our relationship. At the time of this writing we have been together for about three and a half years. The first three years of our relationship was filled with so much beauty but also with a lot of turmoil and pain. When two people get together as a couple who have been through domestic violence, abuse, neglect, and manipulation like we have, it's hard to get to a point of healthy balance.

We also had custody of his niece and nephew for a while as their mom tried to get better. We had considered adopting his nephew but it was just too much for us to handle. It was also unfair to the children. We encountered a great deal of discrimination in many of the systems that we tried to navigate. Even when things got better, we were still discriminated against when we recently tried to get her nephew back in our home. We had learned that he was still not adopted, even though we were told that there was a family for him. This all ended up being lies.

Obviously, I don't want to portray our relationship as always being something that was free of angst and turmoil. We used to have very bad fights. We even broke up once. This had very little to do with us as far as our gender journeys go. For me, it had to do with being abused by past lovers because I was a masculine, female-bodied person. There was only one other partner before David who did not severely abuse me. She saved my life and helped me heal to the point that I could take a break and then be with David.

We also faced a lot of poverty issues and unemployment. During that time I decided to go to graduate school to become a social worker. Currently, I am in my last semester of my two-year program. The first semester was hard on me and my relationship but I am so glad I did it. Now our life, especially the last year, has been great.

David went through several jobs. He started out as a manager in a McDonald's but decided he wanted to try truck driving. We broke up romantically during his truck driving. I felt like he needed the space to discover himself even more than I did. I had started "T" already and he came home to start testosterone and I helped him. It was at that time that I also realized what he had to learn. He had to figure out if he really wanted to transition. He had wavered about it for many years.

Well, fast forward about four months. David was fired from truck driving during Christmas for things that were not really his fault. We both felt he was discriminated against. He came home and told me that he was now going by female pronouns and didn't care if people called him David or Sarah (her birth name). We also decided to get back together.

It was a gradual progression from this stage to the point we are at today. Now Sarah uses her birth name full time and is referred to as "she." However, she is still very much transgender. She seems freer to let out the multiple aspects of her gender. This has helped us in all areas of life including our romantic relationship and sex. Those things always seem to work out better when someone is free to be themselves. She always said that she had felt a lot of pressure to transition. But when she was with me and I stopped contributing to that pressure, she was able to see herself better. Her main reasoning is that she wants a child and wants to be a mom.

That brings us up to our current relationship. Well, as you may have guessed we did not give up on polyamory. As a matter of fact, we have had many partners who have as many labels as there are colors in the rainbow. Some of them are close to us emotionally but we do not have sex with them. Others of them are friends who we have incredible sex with. This point is important in understanding the rest of this story.

The past year has been the most intense and the happiest part of our relationship so far. It was marked, quite appropriately with Sarah coming home from truck driving. It was hard getting used to her living with me again. She had been driving over-the-road for about six months now. I had never really known her as Sarah so even getting my pronouns right was difficult at first. Experiencing that with her gave me a new appreciation for what it must be like for my family and friends who had known me so long as a girl.

It was also difficult for her because I had now been on testosterone for about six months and was really starting to change physically, emotionally, and spiritually. She had always known me as Joe in some capacity. She was the first to tell me that she knew I was transgender. Even so, testosterone does things to a person. My scent was changing, I was getting more hair by the minute, my sex drive increased dramatically and I was a bit more aggressive than before. At the same time I was also somehow calmer.

As time progressed, things gradually improved. We started first by agreeing not to make any assumptions when it came to sex. Instead, the two of us jumped back into our love-making with a renewed passion. Now that both of us had started to really come to terms with our identities, our sexual lives seemed much freer. This was also coupled with the fact that I had been fairly overweight most of my life. I had lost about 100 pounds at this point. These two factors led to some fun discoveries.

Often, nontrans folks think that transitioning is one of the biggest things that has influenced my life so far. Others who have never been overweight think that it is drastic weight loss. However, for Sarah and I, the evolution of our sexuality and spirituality have always been key. All other things seem to influence these two areas. At the same time, they are also the driving force in all of our actions.

At the time that I am writing this, I have not yet had top surgery or bottom surgery. I have only had a hysterectomy and have been on testosterone for eighteen months. My current weight loss is at 130 pounds. When I tell folks this, they seem to think that these things are big feats. For me though, my sense of spirit and my thoughts of myself as a sexual being are what's core to my identity as trans.

See, the further along I go on this path into "manhood" the more I become in touch with the spiritual world and my own place in it. Once I started transitioning I knew that I was called to be a social worker, psychic, and writer all simultaneously. I began doing things like challenging my biggest fears (one of which was surgery). It was as though I had little fear anymore. I still feel this way, even more so.

I have realized that for me, being transgender is a spiritual identity. I strongly feel that I was meant to be a woman for the first twenty-three years of my life. For many years I fought back and forth with myself about transitioning. I went from saying that it wasn't "feminist" to transition—to mutilate my body because I couldn't live in it anymore. Then one day it became clear to me. I went to see the doctor and started taking testosterone. It was my time to finally live life as a transgender male. For me there is no shame in it. I don't blurt it out to everyone I meet but at the same time I have no reason to hide it. The universe made me this way for a reason.

All of this realization brought me into an awakening of sorts. I began traveling down this very spiritual path with Sarah at my side. As this began, life seemed much easier and free. I could actually speak to people with confidence and really see them for who they were inside. I started reading about many different religious and spiritual practices. Among these practices was Tantra and spiritual polyamory.

As I said before, sexuality is another area where we are both greatly impacted. For us, all beings are sexual in some way. Even when we hug or touch someone we are transferring our energy and that is sexual. In the same way, we figured out ways to make love that involved the physical transfer of energy. One night of lovemaking stands out for me as an illustration of this.

We were lying in bed and I was thoroughly frustrated. My mind was filled with thoughts of lacking a penis and not being able to please Sarah and feel it. This is a thought that creeps up for me many times but one that I can usually come to terms with. Well, this drummed up something new in her and she just got on top of me and started kissing me passionately. It was as though she was pouring warm healing energy into me. I just lay there for a minute kissing her back as my pain was slowly being alleviated. Next thing I know, our pants were both off and we were grinding hard against one another. My dick (clitoris) was longer due to the testosterone but not big enough to feel her on top of me. Yet, this was different. So much so that she was grinding against me and ripped off her shirt. I didn't grab her or anything. I just lay there imagining she was riding my energetic cock.

"Just close your eyes and picture me inside you. Breath into my breath and it will produce hot energy," I whispered to her.

So she began riding me faster. As she did this, her breath increased in speed. Then she locked her legs under mine and I wrapped mine around hers. It was like we were one large mass of heat, energy, passion, and emotion. My body was tingling with desire. I had never felt like that in my life. Years of having sex but always feeling strange made it difficult to really be in my body. This was different.

"I should take my shirt off," I said very matter of factly.

She stopped and looked at me funny. See, I rarely, to this day will take off my shirt. If I do, I usually will have a bra on. I don't mind getting touched there sometimes but someone has to really talk to me like my chest is a male chest and I have pecs and so on. This time was different. I longed to be naked with her. It didn't matter what parts I had because in my spirit I had the male body that was right for me.

After explaining this to her, she helped me take off my shirt. Suddenly the heat began to rise again and we moved in unison to the rhythm of our breaths. As we grew faster, hotter, deeper and more passionate, an incredible thing happened. I felt myself having an orgasm with very little stimulation. I held it in for a minute waiting and waiting for what seemed like hours but was really seconds. Next thing I knew she started to orgasm on top of me with such glorious delight. As she was nearing what I thought was her last spasm I grabbed her butt and pushed her down against me. Then I came hard and with a loud grunt of enthusiastic pleasure.

Now, I am not saying that this is always how we have sex. Sometimes our sex just involves mutually touching each other. Often, I will wear a strap-on or penetrate her in other ways. There are also times where I can now get what I naturally have somewhat inside her. I can feel it enough to have an orgasm. The common theme is that we both try to be as spiritually and mentally centered as possible to do this.

See, I find that one of the things that's hard for our nontransgender partners to understand is that for a lot of trans men sex is as much in the brain (and, for many, the spirit) as it is in the body. I have found myself explaining to too many heterosexual and bisexual women that it's different for me because I don't have a large dick like a biological man. For me, I get more pleasure when they are pleasured. I don't want them to just lay there and let me penetrate them. I want them to really get into it. Also, sometimes it is just simply too hard to have sexual intercourse like a "man" and a "woman" do. I appreciate that they see me so much like a male. At the same time, I wasn't born male. I am transgender and so I need my experience as a transgender person validated. I need it to be "ok" that I don't want to have sex in that way right now. This has been difficult for me and the women who are part of my chosen family who I am sexual with.

At the same time, I have also been with two biological men after starting testosterone. They are both great guys who I do consider an important part of my family. The reality is that things are actually a bit easier with them. One of them is legally married to a woman who I also consider part of my family. Sarah and I have been intimate with them in several combinations. We love them, therefore intimacy makes sense.

However, the guy is bisexual and really likes to have me as a person who penetrates him. I have done it only once as I often prefer to be a spectator when more than one other member of my family is involved. It is easier for me as a trans man because sometimes I just cannot connect with my body. Yet, with him, being a top is a lot easier. The particular time where penetration took place we were both very connected. He understood that I couldn't feel it so he guided me and kind of told me what it would feel like had my cock been flesh and blood. It was hot and even though I didn't have an orgasm, it was a wonderful experience.

So, that brings us to guy number two. He is another close person in our lives. We have been seeing him for over six months now. Whenever I mention this man everyone seems to ask me if he has ever "fucked" me in my female parts. The answer to this is yes. He is the only biological man to ever do it, too.

When I tell people that I actually physically enjoy penetration, they freak out. I am very masculine after all. Still, the goddess blessed me with having an extra hole that feels good when penetrated correctly. I don't have any gendered association with this part of my body though. Actually, I often masculinize it by calling it my "manpussy" or "boycunt" and so on. So for me, it means very little to be penetrated except that it is often quite pleasurable. I would trade it for a penis any day but it is what I have and I choose not to hate it. After all, it is all part of the transmale experience in my mind.

Anyway, back to our guy friend. I think what makes him special is the way that he goes about sexuality. He is very bisexual and for him we are the couple that he can do anything with. We have all taken turns being every gender and sexual orientation under the sun. He has also helped me see more closely what it is like to function as a man. I have sat behind him and masturbated him while playing with myself as well. I have knelt behind him and put him inside my girlfriend then guided his motions from behind. We have also had sex where he is penetrating me and I am penetrating my girlfriend. Each time this was very spiritual and energetic. We both get into a somewhat meditative state before we are able to do this for, and with, each other. Our eyes are always closed and we try to match each other's breaths as well as our body movements. While I sometimes have a hard time with this because I will never get to feel what he does, it has also been my most rewarding experience.

I share these sexual stories with you because I strongly feel that it is important to acknowledge that transgender people are sexual beings. We have sexual organs as well as our entire bodies, which feel great pleasure. Taking testosterone makes this even more evident as it increases the sex drive. For Sarah and me, a life without sexuality would not be one worth living. It is one of the greatest gifts that the universe has given us. We as a community of queer and transgender folks must be sure not to desexualize the transgender body and experience.

Before I end I would like to share with you one last thing about my relationship with Sarah. She is my best friend and currently my only life partner. I have many family members but she is the only one who I live with and who I am planning my life with. I proposed to her about a month ago. She said yes but we have our doubts about our union being legally recognized. I live in the United States and the state that I was born in will not change my birth certificate to male without bottom surgery. I am in no place to have this surgery right now and may not for many years. So we cannot get married. If we were, it would only be for the benefits of civil marriage and nothing more.

With that said, we have three major things planned for our future. We plan on finding places where we would like to start careers. Next, we plan on having a beautiful child through artificial insemination. Lastly, we hope to find a woman with whom we can share our life in an attempt to come closer to this thing known as "being complete." Ultimately, we strive for happiness as we continue to fight for our right to pursue those things necessary to attain it.

18

Eternity Fields of Yokatatumba

Vidal Rousso

Two wrongs don't make one right. I've got no sperm. She's got ovaries. I've got ovaries. Two wrongs. Can't make one right.

So, what's the big news? Is it like a big revelation or something? No, not at all. It's not like I'm about to climb that long ladder up to heaven and complain to the old long-bearded biblical daddy-god. First, because I might not find him before my time is up and I fall like a burned moth, my brain cells exploding from the lack of oxygen, and second, he'd kick me right back down. He's got a whole battalion of saints to handle out-of-hand situations. Especially with former Catholics fallen into heathenism.

I just had to be clear and honest. Our story isn't really only about a couple, but rather a threesome, featuring a shadow of the mysterious man to do the man's job where I'm short of it. That's the Doctor Jekyll face of the third. And then there'd be a face of Mr. Hyde this shadow wears, too. A face pushing us to be two rights, even if with a chance that within this particular threesome we might be the ones getting screwed. It's neither a mysterious man nor a woman, nor in-between here; it's an archetypical shadow of the old world, covering not only large expanses in people's cerebral hemispheres, but also whole territories of the globe.

If you want to know what the Old world looks like, go to Latvia. It's a tiny post-Soviet country on the brink of the Baltic sea, where vast brooding forests bathe in the rays of ignorant sun, rivers of wine flow through heterosexually fertile valleys towards the sea, across the beach so beautiful it alone could bring another century of slavery upon its

Trans People In Love

people while ruins of hope sit on the hills, watching in serenity, raising their ancient walls against the horizon. And when you drive
through Riga, the city of Latvia, towards the Old town, you might not
notice, but female cars begrudge female cars, and male cars begrudge
male cars, and nothing in-between is allowed since no car knows then
whose turn is it to do the begrudging. Old town . . . Old town is the
PR's favorite, with a method-acting cock on the spire of St. Peter's
church working on his deeply depressed looks to follow the common
trend, while thinking that nobody's gonna drink the wine of the rivers
straddling him anymore; and the Cathedral, where the hunchback of
Notre Dame awaits in his bell tower for those awake enough to
scramble up and breathe the open air, and look down at the city covered by the existential mist of fear which gives it a gray shade even in
summer. And there, among all these tourist attractions, I got con-
ceived, born, and brought up.

*"What are you writing?" I hear her voice coming into my ear. Si-
lently she has approached me from behind. "Is it that story about us?"*

*I nod. She has washed her hair and its smell is crawling into my
nose, so I catch some strands and plunge my big smeller organ
among them. Looks like she's free. At last, after three working days in
a row.*

*"Fuck the story," I breathe on her skin, moving downwards, to bite
into her porcelain-gentle neck. She lets her fingers loose in my hair,
and I seize them; their joints, their arms, the whole warm body. Carry
her into the bedroom, smashing her knee into the doorpost as usual,
and drop her on our long-suffering, half-broken bed, landing on top
of the little female heap myself.*

*"I'm so horny my brains will blow out," a groan comes while my
tattooed tentacles are kept busy wrapping around the delicate limbs
of my fiancé.*

I don't know if I'm happy now. But I'm a lucky bastard. Whenever
I try to prove the opposite, don't listen. This is a happy story.

I have never known problems with my family. There was nothing
wrong with my childhood (it was a very fortunate one). The trouble
came much later. Not when I found out I had a diagnosis—sounds so
clinical, doesn't it?—a healthy-man-diagnosis of female-to-male
transsexual; that was just a handful of pepper on the whole raw steak.
The steak itself appeared to bother my life in more simple and plain
ways, not all of them irrespective of the transsexuality though.

There's no use to write about them, since this is a happy story. Maybe it will be enough to mention that after my search for a boy or girl-friend, going through years and hands like an old money bill, hands and fists, and brains without a clue, and mouths without a taste, and eyes without a wish (to understand), and loads of cocks and pussies without freedom but with considerable lust, I was gambling for a sum equal to sixty British pounds, striking a deal which doesn't really exist in the real world, only in the movies, to star in an underground torture flick.

Well, I got stolen from my fate. A word, a sentence. Breath. Underbreath. Pride and prejudice coupled with doubt and despair devouring . . . people, people, people . . . running, moving like stirred ants, funny from above and deeply disturbing for those hearing them from underneath; invincible, but fragile, you see them breathing, blinking and you can't hurt them, hurt no one anymore, ever, and words are streaming from their mouths, chatting, injuring, helping, stealing.

Try and find what you want, what you need to hear in this anthill, in this cacophony of sounds and chatter. And when you are in the wrong fraction, don't linger there . . . but how do you know it is the wrong one, if you haven't heard anything else, trying to bounce the words off yourself using the soundproof shield of your family?

And here the girl-queen Luck passed me with her boa. I bumped into a rare kind of friend, just when it was about time and my games with life were getting dangerous once again. He talked differently, in Swedish, in English, in sentences and words I needed to hear, and if not the words, the respect, the help from him, I might have been just about anywhere, but very doubtfully somewhere good.

November has hung up, in a disguise under the name of December. The weather outside is horrible; it's the time in the North when all the shit floats to the surface and depressions react like falcons on anybody moving. It's a Prozac time; everybody saves his brain the way he can, and we too, surrounding ourselves with candles and wine, and Christa's white fluffy blanket in our own trademarked little world. It's like a template for our lives—when the scene outside doesn't fit us we create our own and hide there, never to be found, and I'm her man, and her woman, and her father and son, and a sheep, too, as we drink warm milk with honey, watch arthouse flicks, tickle each other half to death, and do another hundred things just like everybody else. At some point it all ceases to our bodies hibernating under the blanket, dug into the pillows, my nose looking for air, her nose pressed against one or another of my tattoos, the black steed, or the grassland inside a stone triangle on my arm, the one I inked being actually worried about what was awaiting me in the Sweden I was leaving for; the stone therefore was to harden my guts and the grass—to bring a piece of home with me. But life loves irony; it turned all the way around. I have obtained peace here, and some sort of weird wholeness that I've lacked for my whole previous existence.

The beginning of our relationship was as if it would've been tailored according to a perfect custom-made plan. The day I moved to Sweden I started to work there and moved into an apartment Christa had rented for both of us; she hadn't unpacked her stuff either yet. I was white, on the outside, and shaking on the inside. My life changed completely. Among the boxes in a new apartment somewhere in the middle of a new country, with a new girl, new smells and a highly nonunderstandable new language I did probably the only thing I could—I broke into sheer and utter panic.

I don't know if Christa had foreseen this. Probably not. All the way I had come across as a quite sensible and calm guy; probably she had meant it as a welcoming gift instead, but anyways sensing it might be the right moment, she pulled out this doll, the action figure . . .

Man, haven't I forgotten now . . . there was a part of the deal where I was to tell how I found the girl. Well, I would want to say it took place over the Internet, since we managed to wear out the immune system of her computer and this heart of mine while chatting all night long, but that would've never happened. It was during the Stockholm Pride, my first, completely amusing, culture-shocking and wild one, when I was wearing a costume that destined me to not slipping away unseen; her eye didn't miss me either, right at the moment when the said costume was moderately falling apart and I had found asylum in a transvestite tent to fix myself. We didn't talk then, her friend beat her to it, but after a week or two I got a letter from her. And, step by step, many months later our acquaintance and friendship turned into a serious business, resulting in my scheduled arrival on her doorstep.

So, the doll appearing in front of me wore the same costume I had used when we first met. And he looked familiar. Like the only familiar thing I had within the radius of 500 miles. Moreover, he looked unshakably happy all over his dolly face, at which I kept looking, chanting in the back of my head that I haven't just made one of the biggest mistakes in my life, and that the people I cared for back in Latvia will survive, and probably exactly the opposite as well.

There's no memory about sleeping—but that doesn't matter, now does it? No importance whatsoever what exactly we did. All in all I slept, ate, peed—carried out the most basic functions, and also managed to walk and talk, and work well enough so that Christa didn't have to give up her hopes and commit me to an institution or send me back where I came from. Not without a reason: I guess it took me half a year before my past and present lives began to form some sort of a timeline instead of an unshapeable chaos in the middle of which the past reality made the existence of the present one an acid hallucination—vivid but endlessly scary and completely unreal.

So I was zombying myself through life, all ready to go on like that for a while, when my body decided enough was enough, and crashed.

If I knew what a release physical pain would be, I'd have thrown myself at a wall or gotten myself a tropical fever a long time before. There was genuine fear in Christa's eyes, not *of* a hell-tempered, slightly manic, mug-gnawing boyfriend, but *for* him, and something clicked into place. And that was it. There our happy story began; apart from the trouble, of course, which understanding what a great job it had just accomplished, kept us busy for several months nonstop. I'd say the trouble got itself overworked. Nonetheless, it brought us both together closer than Victoria and Prince Albert on their wedding night.

We are still in bed. I moan under her, strap-on rocking heavily inside my ass, and I could swear on my nonexistent moustache I must have a prostate. Even more, I could swear on my remains left after being attacked for verbalizing such a blasphemy, that every man who's never taken it from his woman must be either an ignoramus or a fool. And that's the hard, promiscuous truth. Straight out of a legless, nearly unconscious post-coital life-form frantically running to the bathroom.

And then came the next ordeal. Christa's vacations had just come up so she was leaving for Öland, and I, of course, followed. Her parents own a summerhouse in the Borgholm district, which meant that I was to meet her parents as well. I knew that they weren't having any problems with me, but it wasn't really what I expected. Or, what I could really, truly believe. In Latvia, if your daughter gets together with a transsexual, it is at least ten times worse than if she was fooling around with a bunch of criminals, and if the said transsexual is tattooed, long-haired, and grungy, it makes him . . . pardon . . . her a much more dangerous species, since he . . . sorry, she . . . is not only mentally sick, but maybe stays out of prison just because he . . . uh, again . . . she has the white leaf. (In Latvia if someone says they have the "white leaf" it means they could commit a crime and get into a mental hospital for a period of time or suffer some other mild consequences but would never be fully liable.) If you care one bit about your daughter, you grab your gun and shoot as soon as the transsexual appears anywhere close to the borders of your real estate; it is vitally important he—dammit, what's wrong with me?—she doesn't escape, therefore it is advisable to use a fully loaded automatic. Once you see all her pieces have fallen down and don't move, throw a couple of hand grenades too, only to be sure, since transsexuals, just like homosexuals, are survivors, a bit like cockroaches, and if nothing will be done, soon they will take over the population of the fatherland and the demographic crisis will cause complete and utter depopulation of the country.

The depopulation threat of the Swedish grounds didn't seem to worry Christa's parents though. After some quarter of an hour of waiting on the sandy, long road in the middle of nearly endless fields and several half-hearted attempts to disappear in the high grass on the roadside I felt my body slowly crawling into the poncho and against my willpower, clinging with its little hairs to the inside of the woolen cloth as the expected car appeared at the horizon; the big, black machine came closer and closer, and I was quietly solving the dilemma whether to force my legs towards the road where Christa was waving to the car or let them moonwalk me closer to that grass, but by then the car had already stopped in front of us, and its door opened, and out jumped Christa's mother who gave me a big, warm hug.

Two weeks later. Christa is painting something in the other corner of the room. Still no snow. And that's the thing which hasn't changed. We are unemployed now, both of us, both questioning what to do tomorrow and in ten years. We are both depressed. Sometimes going crazy. At nothing. At each other. At the world. It's easy to find things to go crazy at, when you are unsure, and your guts feel threatened. Who wouldn't? I'm chain-smoking my third cigarette and I do not

smoke. Beware of what I write. No, it's me who should beware, first
and last.

Öland is a place you want to hide once you have found it, so that it
would stay the way it was when you found it, imprinted with high yellow grass of its Arizonian prairies and the beach which, to be honest,
couldn't bring a day of slavery upon its people but every summer evening becomes an open-air movie theater for the most colorful golden
sunsets which look their best in the camera.

And instead of the mist of fear there is a mist of Isla de Muerta,
soft, warm, and so thick you can wrap it around yourself when taking
a skinny dip; neither the air nor water is able to stay cold when you
bathe in this mist. That's where I die, in this mist, and come out of it
newly born, into the sun, hand in hand with my squaw, married by the
water, air, and age-old rocks, the only way a real marriage can be
done. We have eternity in the fields in front of us to walk until we
reach the sunset and fly, burning and free, into it. Our path lies in the
long grass, the prairies of sun, on the long sandy roads between the
villages and red houses . . . rough surface burns the soles of our feet
. . . and we step away from the road when a car passes by, to set a
teepee, to wash in a thunderstorm and teach our children to hear what
a rain worm has to say.

And the car is gone; sun is above our heads and we continue our
way. It's far to go but we are used to walking. I step into the long
grass; my Pocahontas's bare little feet follow mine. She didn't choose
a white man, it's a story told to take money from those who want to
hear it and to buy a lot of needed and unneeded things for it; she chose
a man of her people, me, an outcast from my own tribe, from my own
lands. We are only two people in the middle of the prairie of the sun,
long grass touching our thighs gently and crickets singing to their
women to give birth to more crickets to sing many summers to come
after everybody would be gone from here.

"You," she doesn't say Raphael and I don't say Pocahontas, for
names are only names and right now, right with this breath we want to
talk to each other. We look into each other's eyes. What a great gift it
is that we can see each other; I watch blood pulsating in the vein on
her neck and I watch how she breathes. Our arms wrap around each
other and we stand there, entwined. The sun is going down and the
sky opens up for it, and bursts into flames of a passionate union to

give birth to colors that run all over it. The violet light of the evening is slowly descending over the dry, yellow fields.

"I dreamt once," my woman says, "And I forgot the dream. But my mother reminded me."

We are dreaming now, together with the sky and the meadow and the crickets hiding evening shadows from our eyes.

"There was a vast field of high grass. Someone was walking through it, and I felt it was a man. He had long dark hair; a lot of amulets were tied around his neck—and his wrists; there was only a cloth hiding his hips. He came towards me, his bare feet touching the dry, rustling grass, and he took the sun and put it over my head."

She becomes silent; our fingers touch, we cast a look at each other through the evening light.

"My mother reminded me of my dream when I met you. And then you came to me, wearing the amulet of sun."

Our eyes look the same way as the light becomes darker and darker. The violet dissolves above the grass and through it comes the black shadows of the evening. Still, we sit in the middle of the grass like two charmed stone spirits; the night can never put the darkness over us, for I would see our way in the light of my squaw, but she doesn't know it.

There never will be winter again, I will never work, and that is how the world will end, by drowning in the gray cold slimy mud, bruised against the gravel while trying to pull itself out of this pool of dead leaves and destruction. The wind blows so hard the lamp posts swing with artificial optimism like in a spooky jazz dance, and I put my arm around Christa so she won't be blown away with the branches and umbrellas.

We go to go to the landlord's and leave the old, changed keys. It's ages since we walked this alley; the last time we did, everything was different, and the old feelings with the sharp, bittersweet sting of reminiscences come over me and I stop to linger there. For the sweetness in this torment is more powerful than my constant everyday blues; and suddenly I understand I was happy here, for one year, for real. I had what everybody searches for—happiness. Living and creating, and working I saw the future only better and only upwards, but didn't even crave for that future for I had everything in the present.

Christa's hand is trying to pull me forwards for no being wants to stand still in this weather. I follow, letting the stream of consciousness invade her ears from my opened, wind-raped mouth; she meets mine with hers. The way to the landlord's office is not that long, but this is a story and I can stretch the road like a rubber band if I please; so we talk about the last summer and the summer before, our honeymoon in Öland and about our official honeymoon to come after we are married—no, registered as partners; and that I can't—I absolutely can't understand that we can't be married, for we already are a husband and a wife; we talk about that and how we will get a kid together one day (or night, although days work as well, especially now, when we are unemployed), but then there comes this big revelation that we can't. Unexpectedly, I take it calm, really calm, but it doesn't click. I simply fail to understand. There must be something very wrong with me. After we have been standing outside the landlord's for five minutes and talking, it's time to go inside even if I look like an unemployed serial murderer who has left his Prozac at home.

But one day, sitting in a never-ending autumn train, undisturbed, I turn back and watch graffiti of the perfect happiness imprinted on the gray landscapes behind the window. For there's not much else left to do within this story anyway: Christa became my drug; my safety pill; a friend you dare anything with, long before, and therefore I get to skip the long description of how we grew closer. Besides, that was already mentioned—where I wrote about Victoria's and Albert's wedding, remember? Let's watch the graffiti then. Smell it. Taste, if you dare to jump out of the train and be left behind.

Summer of color, and smells. Blossoming trees. Shea butter melting on Christa's neck. Summer of warm stone, touches of sun, moonlight blended in a lunatic mix with the glare of torches cast over damp night grass and a man and a woman, and a neighbor's kid watching them and their champagne glasses with his chocolate-brown wide eyes. Summer of dirt, ground, soil, hard substance under the feet. Of fear rewound, swallowed by genitals and disintegrated, of dirt naked and natural. Of bodies alive and demanding the fix of their primal hunger, claiming it—taking it on adrenaline, screaming, running naked into the kitchen with only the window separating us from the street and almost getting my nose chopped off by the door Christa tries to close in front of me to save the neighbors—or us—I didn't really understand; or being thrown down to the floor if it was too late and I had already managed to stroll into the kitchen. Not that I'm complaining; the throwing on the floor is always nice, you keep coming back for some. However, if during the most paranoia-ridden years of my life the need to pass ruled my whole existence, it wasn't the case anymore; I wanted a chance to go into my kitchen in my underpants like any other man, and get a cup of tea.

Like any other man, huh. What would any other man do upon finding two boobs on himself, transvestite tendencies already given? I managed to sully our family image in front of both our neighbors forever. Bad luck, yeah, and the heat, that's what was to blame; but how could I have known that when I jumped out of the apartment into the back garden in women's clothing, both neighbors would be out there in their gardens? Even the one to the right of us who never comes out, was out, amen.

The neighbors took it well; a score to them since sure enough I wasn't wearing any socially correct female outfit. Rather something like . . . uh . . . trashy Caribbean grunge with sexual overtones? Anyway, when I had jumped out there like a promiscous Malecón drag queen on the streets, the men from both directions checked the drag queen out, and then there was no use jumping back in, now was there?

We have fucked again. Well, what else is there to do when you are both unemployed and the creative flow refuses to flow anywhere except for in a circle, repeatedly, until you get nauseated and run to the toilet. We have fucked and are lying on our crimson sheets next to each other, two pale figures, naked, sweaty, exhausted. What bliss. Peace.

"*What did you do?*"

A voice, probably in my head. I open my eyes and he stands there, at the bedside table, the little gray bulge-eyed psychotherapeutic counselor of the Yokatatumba National Health Service.

"*I had sex.*"

The counselor's ears start growing, getting ready for listening, but I don't feel too talkative, if I were given a choice I'd rather turn over and fall asleep. After I keep silent for several minutes he speaks up again.

"*Are you comfortable?*"

What kind of dumb question is that? Doesn't he see?

"*How do you feel about your body?*"

"*Relaxed. Post-orgasmic. I don't quite feel my legs all the time . . .*"

"*That's not really what I mean,*" *he cuts in.* "*She touched you. You are naked. How do you feel? Many transsexual men feel like keeping a t-shirt on before they have transitioned . . .*"

"Oh. Great. She touches me all she likes, I don't have to be afraid she will start thinking I'm a girl."

"But how does it feel for you? Being in the wrong body?"

I crawl out of the bed and go stand in front of the mirror built into our wardrobe, on the way almost trampling on the counselor. He's little and gray, hard to see. "Come here. Is it a wrong body if it's mine? Look," *I slide my hands over my chest and his eyes bulge out a little more,* "Use a little imagination . . . I have a male chest. Thighs. My ass . . ." *I turn to the side.*

"Don't you long for a dick?" *he has opened his notebook, little and gray. This must be a crucial question.*

"I have read volumes about the SRS online," *I sit down on the carpet, and now our eyes are on the same level.* "If I can't feel what a man feels when he fucks his woman—I don't need it."

"I agree both metoidioplasty and phalloplasty are not perfect yet," *he nods, writing something down.* "But, as you have probably read, you don't have to choose them. Many FTM transsexuals are completely happy with hormone therapy, mastectomy, and hysterectomy. How do you feel about cutting your hair?"

"You touch my hair and you'll be dead."

Suddenly the little gray one is gone. Never knew they might be so quick. The better for me, maybe I will get my sleep now. Still, returning to the bed I spot a corner of his notebook between sleeping Christa and the wall, and there he is, hiding behind his papers.

"Oh, really, man, do you think I would kill a psychotherapist? You stay clear of me and I stay clear of you, and all is gonna be fine. Now get out of my bed and away from my woman!"

He crawls out of the bed, trying to keep as far from me as possible, almost stumbling over the pot where our Areca palm stands.

"Can I ask you a couple more questions?"

"Go on," *I put my head down on the pillow. There's moonlight on the floor. Sometimes we sit up on such nights and watch it, in complete peace and serenity. As if we could be stolen by the moonlight and dropped somewhere to sail the seven seas, without borders, work permits and customs' officers.*

"What do you think about the transition then?"

"Absolutely nothing."

Christa, turning around, puts her palm on my stomach and I cover it with mine. It feels safer to talk to that gray counselor now, when my girl is so close. "You are so completely obsessed with my body soon you will crawl into my mirror. Why do you think that a female body makes me female and a male body would make me male? I am male. Why do I need to cut myself?"

Suddenly I notice that I sound like a Native American and the counselor's eyes are bulging out with enormous capacity, genuinely trying to understand.

"See, I'm male. And I don't hate my female body. It works, and it's mine. But I am male, and I don't want to cut myself or swallow pills just in order to get people to admit I am who I am. Understand?"

He nods, as all good Yokatatumba National Health Service psychotherapists do, and continues, "Are you really sure you are transsexual? Could you explain a little how can it be . . ." At this point Christa turns in the bed and her hand, before peacefully lying on my stomach, now makes a circle in the air and catches him on the mouth. I see no point in continuing tonight, so I don't answer and close my eyes. When I open them again, he's gone.

I touch my crotch under the blanket. It's flat, as usual, hairy. There's no cock, of course. Goodness, what a pleasure it must be to father a child. What a pleasure it must be just to come inside a woman . . . But, when I'm with her, I don't really care about those things. They pass me like a breeze of wind, touching lightly, and giving way to other thoughts, more important thoughts. Thoughts about stuff that might and can happen, not about what can't. This is a happy story, do you see it now? Do you? Now?

It has taken years until I let myself shake off the old world and be a genuine wrong instead of a fake right; and it took people who see me for who I am so that I could become me. It takes some guts sometimes, but without these people and, most importantly, Christa, it might take too much guts. And if none are left, how would I survive, when the guts are a vitally important part of the digestion system?

I cast a caress with my eyes over Christa's sleeping face, turn my back to her, so that our asses press against each other, and close my eyes. It's snowing outside. At last.

19

My Husband Had a Sex Change—Shit Happens

Erica Zander

If the title gives you the impression that this piece was actually written by my partner, this is not correct. It could have been though, had she only written the book that quite a few of our friends suggested and for which I claimed this title in her name. Now that it's obvious she never will, I thought I'd better use it myself before someone else snatches it from under our noses.

This said, it should be obvious that I'm a post-op male-to-female transsexual, she is my former wife, and we still live together. We have also chosen to be quite public with our situation, to give Swedish transsexualism a couple of —at least quite—ordinary faces.

WAY BACK WHEN

For this to make sense I suppose we should go back to August 1, 1970, when we first met outside a pub in Wexford, Ireland. I was hitchhiking around the country with a friend of mine and she was on a day-trip from Wales, where she spent the summer improving her English. We were both seventeen. With her living in the south of Sweden and me in Stockholm, our contact was limited to a few long letters—making her boyfriend go mad with jealousy and her to gradually wonder who I might be, behind my facade of immature innocence.

Basically I think she was right. Born late in the year and a late bloomer at that, I probably was quite innocent but there was also this female side to my personality that I had begun to express openly in town, a couple of years before. Getting to know other trans persons, going to gay clubs and so on, inevitably added a not-all-that innocent note, and when, two years later, we met again, she told me, after our first night together, that "I'm simply not letting you go this time." So far she has kept her promise for almost thirty-five years, through joys and sorrows, good and bad, happiness and pain.

As for my being trans, I did tell her about my—so I thought—transvestism a few months into our relationship. This didn't worry her much, and on our very first New Year's Eve she joined me at a private gay and lesbian party, for which I dressed as a woman.

In 1974 she moved to Stockholm—"temporarily"—and late in December we moved in together. My dressing as a woman was soon a natural part of not only our daily life, but also that of our friends. This was also when my media career started with a number of newspaper, magazine, and radio appearances on the subject of gender issues.

Now and again T asked if eventually I might opt for a sex change but of course I said no—mainly because I was so totally into girls. According to the "experts" of the time this meant that I was not and could never be a transsexual, and when society tells you that you don't exist, it's all too easy to believe that they are right. I'm amazed, though, that neither one of us wondered why I dressed in jeans and t-shirts when all the other trannies liked to dress up in frills and lace . . . and why, a couple of years later, I started going to lesbian clubs.

In June 1975 we got married and I should have been seriously worried when this caused me to decide, on a not-all-that-conscious level, that I would not consider getting female hormones for at least four more years. Where did I even get the idea? Throughout all this, our sex life flourished. Considering what would eventually happen I suppose this is quite strange, but obviously we found ways of expressing ourselves so that male or female didn't really matter. Another part of the explanation probably is that we both always liked sex and were never shy about it.

FAMILY

Three years later our eldest son was born, and the following summer, in a tiny tent in Italy, I told my wife that I had to find a doctor who would prescribe me estrogen, not even for a second remembering that this was an idea I put on hold four years earlier. My argument for this strange wish was that the hormones might make me feel more "whole" when not explicitly dressed as a woman. She didn't seem overly worried.

Finding this doctor was easy enough, with the Stockholm medical team for the treatment of transsexuals, but it took me fifteen months of regular meetings—and one cracked-up male psychiatrist at that: "I don't ever want to see another transsexual again!"—to convince them that in spite of my not being properly classified as transsexual (TS), I needed this prescription to continue "being" on a meaningful level. When finally I succeeded, two months after the birth of our second son, I was the first one ever in Sweden, and I wouldn't be surprised if I'm still—twenty-six years later—the only one who ever did.

In spite of the physical changes being so small that I could always pass for a man on the beach, and quite a fit specimen at that, the hormones made me feel much more here, now, and in-myself, so when two years later, after a winter and spring with fading dividing lines between my male and female personae, I suddenly stopped dressing as a woman, literally from one day to the next, I believed this to be a result of my having found a working balance between the two. A more fundamental part of the explanation was probably that my two closest trannie friends—androgynous jeans and t-shirt girls like myself—had recently realized they were both transsexuals, and were now heading for legal and physical womanhood. As this obviously wasn't for me . . .?

I cut my hair quite short, took the rings out of my ears, and settled down to being an ordinary husband and father—a role I can honestly say I was pretty good at. As for my twenty-five years of consciously wanting to be a girl, I now considered myself to be "a former trans." Not for a moment did I entertain the idea that I would stop taking my hormones, though. So obvious was it to me that this new mental balance was all their making.

The only one who didn't believe me was my wife; to her it was just a matter of time when my female side would surface again. In a way she probably missed "Erica," associated as she was with friends and parties, but I'm sure it was also about being quite queer herself. Not all that easy to understand, though, with queer theory still fifteen years in the making.

AND SEVEN BAD ONES

After seven nice years of "former transdom" I got my first serious warning that T might well be right. One lovely spring day in Munich, alone with a cool beer at a sidewalk café, I decided to write a letter to one of my transvestite (TV)-gone-TS friends. Before I knew what happened I had put down the words "Could it be that I'm a transsexual after all, but just didn't dare to see it?" In spite of this quite upsetting incident I didn't have a clue what was going on when I started growing my hair long again, relocated a couple of old piercings in my ears, and then gradually added new ones.

Over the next seven years—it does sound quite biblical, but really was the way it happened—I spent most of my business trip evenings alone, drinking too much beer and writing quite confused letters to my friend. But when T asked if I was still convinced that my trans side was fast asleep I said yes, without even a note of hesitation. Secretly I did dress up as a woman on a couple of occasions to make sure. It felt quite nice but "did" nothing for me, so I soon took my skirt and bra off again to get back into my more comfortable jeans.

Hard as these years were, I still thought that life was quite ok, but in early 1997 I was so distant and unreachable that our sons decided to talk to their mother about it—"Dad isn't happy"—and a few months later T seriously considered leaving me because there wasn't enough left of me to have a relationship with.

Just the other day, when this piece was almost finished, I decided to sort one of my numerous piles of papers, and I happened to find some photos from that time. The look in those eyes seriously scared me—or rather the lack of a look; there simply was no one home.

One reason for my mental absence was that I spent quite a lot of time on an extensive letter to my doctor, trying to convince him to supply me with more efficient hormones. I still didn't have a clue as to why, but when he simply said, "ok," I was more relieved than I should have been, considering my "former trans" status.

A few days later, and only the day after my eldest son's gradua-tion—coincidences, anyone?—I went to Paris on a business trip, ritu-ally administered my first dose of the new drug, went out in town, suddenly realized that I had stumbled upon the gay quarters of Marais, spotted this nice gay bookstore, walked in, found a stand with lesbian magazines, had a look at these—only from curiosity, mind you; used to go to lesbian clubs, remember?—and literally in a frac-tion of a second realized that I never was this hetero guy "who should have been a woman," but a homosexual woman with obvious body problems.

Interestingly enough "lesbian" was my first choice, with "trans-sexual" being only my second shocking realization that day. And it happened so fast that I got nauseous. Also, it honestly wasn't until this day that I realized what my subconscious had been trying to tell me with my—by then—waist-length hair and numerous earrings.

NEW STATE OF THINGS

My new hormones worked wonders; Already the next morning ev-ery cell in my body tingled and in a couple of weeks' time my tits were all swollen—more so than at any time during my first sixteen years on estrogen. Regrettably not having told my wife that her "for-mer trans" husband intended to start growing tits for real, I did have big problems during that summer's American mid-west family vaca-tion, having to come up with a reasonable explanation as to why I avoided all the campsite pools.

By now it should have been obvious, even to me, where I was head-ing, but I still didn't understand the implications. When some three months later I finally dared to bring my revelation up with my wife, I still clung to this lifeline of "really" being a transsexual but not hav-ing to do anything about it—just nice to finally know. This was during a lovely fall weekend at our summer house—red and yellow trees, blue sky and crisp air, long walks in the gentle September sun—and when I told her, lying on a worn sheepskin in front of the fireplace, she looked warmly at me for a few long seconds, and then said, as the most natural thing, that, "It makes sense. Of course you're a lesbian."

With our sons studying in other parts of the country we saw no rea-son to tell them until the following spring when things had settled down a bit. As nothing much had happened since I first talked to T about it, we couldn't tell them much more than my "really" being a transsexual. This didn't worry them much. Why should it, if nothing would really change?

As for my new drugs, they also improved our sex life in that they heightened my sensitivity to touch immensely, opened up a direct electrical circuit between nipples and genitals, and raised my orgasms to heights I could never have dreamed of, involving my entire body, from the tips of my toes to my ears. Sorry guys, you do miss out on something beautiful!

Paris again: We spent a week there on our way by train to Barcelona the following summer, visited some of the lesbian bars I had found the year before, and when our youngest son had joined us we went for a picnic in the park beneath the Pont Neuf bridge. This was where I realized that of course I'm a transsexual for real and had to do something about it. I did not tell T in so many words, but merely hinted at my insights and spent the following sleeper train nights reading a German transsexual anthology I had found in a Paris fetish shop.

Back in Stockholm I had to face the fact that at the time the Swedish capital didn't have a specialist TS team, but with a little help from my friends I found a psychiatrist willing to see me "to listen to my story and give me some advice." I guess you realize what happened? I sat down in her chair, locked my eyes on hers and heard myself say that, "I want to have a sex change." And to make sure I wouldn't have to lie my way through the process I boldly added that, "If I get an ok, I will probably end up as a full-blown lesbian." When this woman calmly replied, "Before we meet next time I will have to get a copy of the guidelines for evaluation of transsexual patients—and as for your eventual lesbianism, we're really here to talk about your gender, not your sexuality," I could have kissed her!

LIFE AT HOME

My wife knew I was seeing this psychiatrist in relation to my gender identity but claims that I never told her what was really going on. I have no excuse; I guess I simply thought that it was all obvious, and when my doctor and one of her psychologist colleagues asked T to join me for a discussion about my probable sex change, she was quite upset with me for a day or two. That really was it, so I guess that deep within she did know all along. Or maybe I should rather say "feared the worst but hoped it couldn't be this bad?" Strangely enough, she didn't really give much thought to this new turn of events, but quite calmly decided that, "You are the love of my life, and of course I can't leave you because of a sex change. I'm sure we can work this out." Not that it was always easy, but beneath her sadness, sorrow, frustration, and anger, this really was her fundamental belief, and most of the time our life together was nothing short of great. Her conviction was true even to the point where she saw our enforced divorce—no married people can legally change sex in Sweden—as more of a catastrophe than the fact her husband was going to be a woman, society deserting us when we needed their support the most.

We did vent our mutual frustration, though, by bringing this outdated law up for public debate. After numerous newspaper headlines to the effect that "Society forces them to apply for a divorce," and my formally granted audience with the legal committee of the Swedish Parliament, it really was no big deal to actually sign the papers for our application. We had caused quite a turmoil in this little pond and definitely helped pave the way for soon-to-be sex/gender neutral marriages in Sweden. Our divorce was also made much easier by the fact that it was formalized just after we celebrated twenty-five years of marriage.

By this time I had been going to work as a woman for three months, but paradoxically returned to, if not a male state, then at least androgyny in the evenings and over the weekends, so at home nothing much really changed. With our sons still being away from home—the youngest one as far away as Chicago—we saw no reason to tell them what was going on until just before I started dressing as a woman for work. Also, with more earrings and even longer hair, it wasn't that they could forget about their father's slightly strange inclination. When we did tell them, it was in a carefully worded letter, so as to give them a chance to think things over before they had to say something clever about it. In spite of the graveness of the message, they both replied almost immediately, in e-mails more lovely than we could even have dreamed of. Love you guys!

A WOMAN

In February 2001 I was summoned to The Committee for Forensic Psychiatry, Social and Medical Legal Questions to get my verdict, which turned out to be, "We hereby conclude that you are of the female sex" and I returned home with a feeling of emptiness rather than relief. Was this all there was to it? T suggested that we go to our favorite pub to celebrate, but when some guys came on to us she started to cry.

A month later I had a new name and social security number, and spent several weeks trying to sort all the paperwork out in regard to insurance, savings, my monthly pay and bills—for a couple of months, it really was quite a feat to keep track of where my money was—passport and driver's license, the medical system, ownership of car, apartment and summer house, my retirement money and so on.

It was hard to accept the fact that my surgery would be postponed for a couple of months because of summer vacations, but all in all this was probably perfect for our relationship. In May we went to Greece for "a last vacation with my husband"—that is, I traveled as an androgynous man, in a name which didn't officially exist anymore and with a legally obsolete passport.

We then spent a July week in Turkey as two women, one of whom would not have passed a body search, and going to the beach in a ladies swimsuit with nylon panties tucked into the cups sure was a challenge. On the other hand, the way we were invited with open arms into the Turkish women's world was simply magnificent!

August 20, 2001 saw my rebirth as the woman I should always have been. T realized I would probably be only half-conscious that day and didn't visit me until the following evening. I almost cried when she handed me a pair of lovely earrings with the words "for having been such a courageous girl."

Post-op sex was a matter of treading gently on previously unknown ground. First of all, my brain had to sort the new plumbing and wiring out, which felt like very slow electric currents crisscrossing the lower part of my abdomen at irregular intervals. It didn't take long though for the map to be perfectly rewritten and for all the strange phantom sensations to cease, such as having a perfect hard-on where now there was no penis, or wanting to scratch an itch without knowing exactly where it was.

Orgasms? Some eight and a half months post-op I suddenly "found" the first one but it was to be another four years before I could quite accurately feel when I would be capable of having one; it was like there had to be a sufficient amount of pent-up sexual energy for an orgasm to be possible. It's also obvious that the right hormonal balance is a must. My doctor had warned me that eventually I would need testosterone injections as well and when, three years post-op my orgasms got to be much more elusive, he proved to be right; testosterone paradoxically is necessary to have rewarding sex even for a female.

MORE MEDIA COVERAGE

Now let's take a small step back, to the Stockholm Pride inauguration. Our biggest national daily newspaper wished to run a feature story on something other than the ordinary gay gal or guy. I was their pick of the day, and the bold headline claimed that, "The State forced her to file for a divorce." A couple of days later I received an e-mail from Swedish TV celebrity, Malou von Sivers, to the effect that, "I have interviewed the likes of Ingmar Bergman, Nelson Mandela, Kofi Annan, and Isabella Rossellini and now I would very much like to meet you."

Her timing couldn't have been more perfect; we met for the first part of the interview a mere week before my surgery, and then again a month post-op. When the half-hour program was broadcast in early December it seated 10 percent of Sweden's population in front of their TVs ... and Malou was already busy with the sequel. This full-hour version, featuring both of us, our relationship and family life, was televised in December 2002, and obviously made the viewers realize that even transsexuals are quite ordinary people, leading ordinary lives. Drunkards outside our liquor store asked me if "everything is ok? Are people nice to you?," and a bunch of beer-happy thirty-year-old guys on a Gothenburg tram—"now or never I will get a punch on the nose!"—commented on "the very nice program" and wished me a happy life. Four years later we are still met with warm smiles from unknown passers-by in the street.

PROS AND CONS

In a way my eventual transsexualism was a relief to T, in that it explained why I had always been so focused on women—more frequently than not sticking to an old or new female friend at even the most ordinary of dinner parties. This also made it easier for her to understand my need for female company in general, lesbians in particular, and she willingly accompanied me to gay pubs, dyke clubs, launch parties for feminist magazines, and so on. What always took me by surprise was that afterwards she was frequently disappointed, upset, or even outright angry with me.

In a broader perspective this is fully understandable, but from my emotional point of view it was a total denial of my now obvious right to be both a woman among women and a lesbian among lesbians. This being what I had longed for since childhood, her reaction hurt terribly and I simply couldn't understand it.

As for sex, my first optimistic initiatives were regarded with suspicion. She didn't know how to handle this strange situation—identifying as a heterosexual but intending to live in a sexual relationship with another woman—and it was to be ten weeks before she even felt my new crotch through my jeans, and another eight months before she dared to touch me for real. This unique chance to feel a trans cunt didn't tempt her much, but when finally she dared to put her fingers inside, it was only to find that it felt exactly like her own—neither scary nor exciting.

Also, only the day before she had her first look at my pussy, claiming that she needed to search me for ticks. Soon a smile spread over her face. "It looks just like the real thing. Actually it's quite cute!"

Starting from here she soon got to be quite fond of my new body, especially my small but undeniably real breasts, and she was not happy when I gave in to my doctor's advice to accept the implants that were part of the Public Health Care deal. His argument was that looking as "normal" as possible would help me in everyday life, and fifteen months after my genital surgery—when the full effects of testosterone depletion should be obvious—I had them quite substantially enlarged. Of course he was right. Looking more like an average woman of my size added substantially to my sense of being genuine, and also is a must for daring to enter all female domains like ladies' dressing rooms, showers, saunas, and the like.

GOING SOUR

T didn't like my new breasts at all, in that they stressed my new status as something other than "my former husband." In spite of this, she did try really hard, and in time got to be more interested in having sex than I was. In light of her still being quite stable in her heterosexual identity, and my being a dyke, this really was quite hard to fathom.

November 2004—was this when everything took a turn for the worse? There was this unexpected offer of a limited exchange program within the company I worked for, and when I realized that perhaps I could spend three months at our Sydney office, this seemed like a lovely chance to finally get around to visiting Australia. I immediately sent T a text message to this effect. She, on the other hand, was at an important conference, and interpreted this message as being my first step towards life as a single woman; I was very happy, she was not, and we did not understand each other's points of view.

After I got my ok from Sydney, the rest of that winter and spring were not much fun, to say the least; T, who was always a keen traveler, had to be persuaded to join me for a two-month vacation down under, and throughout our six weeks of extensive travel in Australia and New Zealand she persisted in this being nothing but the beginning of our actual separation—the legal one having been forced on us five years before. Then there was this traumatic discussion in the car stemming from my provocative claim that sex between us might actually be more complicated for me than it is for her, on our 300 mile return trip across the wonderful red deserts between Uluru and Alice Springs.

AUSSIE SHIELA

In spite of it all I really was quite a good girl after T left me, in mid August, to return to Sweden. What I did, though, was try to find the fastest way possible into Sydney's dyke world, and by a combination of luck and determination I quite innocently walked into the Dykes On Bikes Sunday hangout only four days after T left me alone on the other side of the world.

I do admit to having forgotten that making friends really takes quite some time, and this incredible coincidence proved to be my lucky card in that I left the place that evening with an invitation for the following week's traditional three days at a bush resort. I rented the biggest Harley I could find for this grand event, spent a lovely weekend in total female and dyke seclusion, started up what proved to be a couple of long-lasting friendships, and had Sunday and Wednesday evenings cut out for the rest of my stay for beer and pool at two different venues.

To me this was all a matter of belonging, of finally having found my kin and being accepted in my own right. I really had been quite worried about the Australian biker dykes' possible trans prejudices, but when president Janet had a close look at me and whispered "Are you transgendered?" so that no one else in the bar could overhear, and I replied, "It says female in my passport, I have a female body, and I'm a hundred percent lesbian, so does it really matter?," she said simply, "I guess not," and never again broached the subject.

There was also Pam's Blue Mountains tour and a barbecue in her garden, late-night pub talks with Laura, lunch with Lucy and Kelly in Bondi, lunch with Katherine, lesbian strip clubs and bisexual cabarets, volunteer work as a gay movie festival orderly and late-night Sleaze Party marshal, and then another biker dyke Saturday, which led to my meeting a totally different bunch of bikers and new friends Sue and Duane, who offered to take me to Snowy Mountains for another amazing weekend. I also managed to leave a lasting impression behind, with a lovely Lesbians On The Loose (LOTL) interview hitting the streets only days before I left Australia.

To me this was all a matter of belonging, and to try to avoid misunderstandings and unnecessary suspicions I wrote long weekly e-mails to my colleagues and family telling them everything, which regrettably worked the wrong way. When I returned home, a Sunday morning in late October, T had decided to leave me for good. I had sensed that this was coming and half expected to find my stuff piled up outside our door, but instead met a woman who looked at me with surprised curiosity in her eyes and a tentative but warm "Hi." It was a strange moment there in our hallway; she wasn't ready to leave yet.

2006

2006 started off on a very nice note when T agreed that—after twenty-three traumatic years without one—the boys were now old enough for me to buy a new motorbike. This I did in late January—a lovely 1100cc burgundy metallic Moto Guzzi California and when summer arrived it proved to be the warmest and sunniest for decades. This finally convinced T that motorbikes really are a lot of fun so in late August she bought herself an old 650cc Guzzi Florida—without ever having driven a bike. When she took to it like she was born on a motorbike, this fundamentally changed her self-image, and she also admitted that my sex change was to blame for this sudden impulse to buy one of her own; to be a pillion rider with her husband was ok, despite her being the most enthusiastic car driver in the family—but with another woman? Not ok.

All in all it proved to be one of our best years ever, and this in spite of the clouds accumulating on the horizon. For her it was a matter of having to accept that life with a husband-turned-girlfriend wasn't as easy as she had imagined. This was partly due to the fact that she had been too optimistic about our chances to begin with, but also to her unexpected conviction that by now I really am a woman, and that there was simply nothing left of her former husband.

For me it was all about this new woman having been neither a teenager nor a female in her twenties, thirties, and forties. I was born at forty-eight, with an almost insatiable need to compensate for all this, and also to find out who I really am, outside of the relationships, work, and so on that Erica simply inherited from her male predecessor. I needed new friends, and also a chance to be as ordinary a woman as possible with the old ones. This naturally meant having closer and more "girl style" intimate relationships with other women—and some of them being lesbians, T did not want to see the inevitability of this development. I do understand her position but regrettably there's nothing I can do about it; I simply can't afford to wait any longer unless I want to end up as a bitter old woman. This, needless to say, was not what I envisioned.

UNDERSTANDING

In early January 2007, something changed dramatically in our relationship. Gone was the frustration, the silence and/or nagging. Instead, there was nothing but warmth, kindness, caring, and really seeing each other. At first I was afraid that T had blocked it all out, to pretend that everything was just fine—taking away all my chances for continued discussions about another future—but one long, beautiful morning in bed we came to some lovely conclusions; probably we have been almost perfect for each other, complementing each other's personality traits and so making up a strong and mainly positive relationship. This worked as a solid foundation which helped us through tough times, both in the world around us and on an individual level. Neither one of us would have managed to become who we are today had it not been for our life together.

At the time of this writing, there are hints at our not living under the same roof when this book is published, but also that we will remain close friends for the rest of our lives. Could it be otherwise after thirty-five amazing years together? I hope not . . .

20

Things of His

Jordy Jones

Some things that were His: a belt, a chair, a hanky, a snapping cock-ring, a collar. And me. With the exception of the hanky, which is red bandana-print cotton, and me, all are black and made of leather. I'm leather, but white. Or rather, I'm one of those light pinkish-brown tones that are usually called white. But that doesn't matter. Or rather, it does because it always does, but it is not what I want to talk about here, now, to you. A black person (or someone who is what is usually called black) has said that different readers create different readings. That's so simple, so obvious, that it verges on idiocy to even mention it, but since we forget it so often, and with such obstinacy, I repeat it just as often and just as stubbornly.

I mention it here because I want for a moment, before proceeding, to consider my reader. I don't know you, or rather, I don't know who you are. I don't want to make assumptions about what you do or do not know or what languages (and I do not mean national or ethnic languages) you speak. The one thing that I do know is that you are reading a volume on love among trans people. (That sounds so exotic, so anthropological. Don't forget to take your camera!) And that is all. After that, the reading is yours. Like I was His. Let me explain, then, what I mean.

As a kid I made no sense. I made some to myself, and to my close friends, but I was (made) aware that I made little to others. I did not fit easily into common categories. As a little girl, I played with (other) little boys. We played the ritualistic games of little boys, compromising ourselves and humiliating one another and standing as witnesses so that the group would be cohesive. Girls weren't allowed. Among other crimes, they told. But I was explained away with "Jordy's balls are inside." And I kept expecting them to drop.

At twelve, I was (mis)taken for a(nother) boy by some boys I spent the summer with on the beach, battling with sticks and jumping from cliffs onto the sand and into the water. At fourteen, I went to a new school where girls who befriended me were taunted with "Lezzie!" and boys who did were called "Fag!" I became aware that I queered those around me—whichever sex they happened to be.

At eighteen I gave blowjobs to the guys in the back patio of The After Dark, a gay bar in Monterey, California. I didn't know (or care) who (or what) they thought was sucking their cocks. I doubt they cared either. I was good. At twenty, I had a serious discussion with my first real boyfriend (who liked other guys but was reluctant to carry that stigma) about whether or not our relationship made him gay. We decided that somehow, it did. After that, when people asked me, "What are you?" (as they often did) I replied, only half-joking, that I was "a freak of nature." I had heard of Renée Richards and Christine Jorgensen, but had no idea that things could go the other way, too. When I found out, I also found out that the existing clinics were "not in the business of creating homosexuals." If I wanted to transition, I was expected to like the ladies, to have a girlfriend, to want a wife. I didn't. Instead I had a gang of drag queens and ambiguous perverts who were as off the charts in their tastes as I was in mine. That was 1992. The following year I met a trans man who had access to black market testosterone and that is how I started my transition.

By the time I met (really met) Alan, I was eight years into transition. I looked all right. No one asked anymore, "What are you?" Clothed, I was cute enough: no great beauty, but no troll either. Nice eyes and a great ass. So when He met me, there was no reason for Him to think that I was anything other than what I appeared to be. I had seen Him around for years, and we had even met once or twice. San Francisco may be a world-class city, but it is also a very small town. I had seen Him on stage at the SF Eagle, the City's main leather "show" bar, running this or that benefit, usually for The AIDS Emergency Fund (AEF), His favorite charity. He was always cool and charming on the mic, very suave with a British voice like honey. An incorrigible flirt. I knew who He was. He was famous in certain circles. I was famous in certain circles. We were famous in the culturally local sense that a friend of mine has dubbed "gaymous." Our circles overlapped, but there was (at least) as much separation as there was intersection. So, when the time eventually came for me to "tell Him" I had no idea whether or not He already knew.

This is how that happened. At the time, I was on the board of directors of The San Francisco Pride Parade and Celebration Committee—"Pride" for short. That's the group that puts on the big annual parade that provokes such eyebrow-raising and tongue-clicking among people who spend too much time looking for sin outside of their own souls. Pride always selects an array of honorees, and special guests and marshals and grand-marshals: it's as arcane as the Elks, really. Alan had been selected as leather marshal that year. He was to ride in the parade in a special car and wave to the cheering crowds. You know the wave? The parade wave: a slow rotation of the right hand, a slow rotation of the left hand, then fingers to the forehead and up. I've heard it described as: "Lightbulb. Lightbulb. Tiara." The weeks leading up to the main event are filled with parties. Honorees and marshals, and celebrities and special guests and politicians and board members are all expected to attend, and to mix, and to pose for the press. So we "met" in the hors d'oeuvres line over crudités and puff pastries.

He started by talking about me—not to me—in front of me. Staring at me, looking directly into my eyes, He quietly told Peter (a mutual friend) that this boy right here had a really succulent ass. Alan was like that. Things that no one else could have pulled off, He could. Words, that if anyone else had said would have been outrageous in a bad way, were from Him, because of His style and grace, outrageous in the best way possible.

"Are you two . . . lovers?" he purred.

"Ummm . . . no?"

"You look like a very horny boy."

"Ummm . . ."

My friend Christopher, who was another in the ever-expanding array of annual good, great and grand-marshals was draped over me, nibbling at a grape cluster and watching the scene unfold. Alan's beautiful heavy-lashed dark eyes danced with mischief. I turned pink. He smiled and turned His back to me. A red cotton hanky peeked out of His left-hand back pocket. He was tall and well-built, not young but strong. He wore boots, big ones. His hands were huge. I looked at the hanky. I can read code.

"Who's that?" Christopher drawled. Alan and Peter had moved out of earshot.

"Alan Selby," I replied.

Christopher shook his head, not recognizing the name.

"You know. Alan Selby? Mr. Selby? Mr. S?

"Of . . .?"

I nodded and Christopher looked suitably impressed.

"He's leather marshal this year."

"Oh . . ."

Two, three, now four years later, I'll sometimes put a boy (not every boy) on his knees. I'll hold a certain very old, very strong, well-worn black leather collar in front of his face while I tell him a story. It goes like this:

> A long time ago, in London, England, there was a man who was a clothier. He was in the business of manufacturing fine men's suits. There was also a boy, good with his hands, who worked with leather making all sorts of accoutrements. They met and the boy became the man's boy. To mark that occasion, the boy made a collar, which he subsequently wore. They moved to San Francisco, where they opened a shop making and selling leather goods. In the early days of the plague, the boy died. Over the years many other boys wore the collar, including two other special ones, both of whom the man also buried. And then, I wore it. When the man died, it came to me. As a historical piece, it "should" be at the Leather Archives and Museum in Chicago with most of the rest of His leather. But He wanted me to have it and He wanted me to use it. The boy who made it was Pete Vanston, the man he wore it for was Alan Selby and the shop they opened together was Mr. S. Leather.

I watch the boy's eyes get big, and I push the collar close to his nose. He inhales deeply, his eyes always dropping closed, his mouth usually dropping open. It smells of leather and sweat and steel and testosterone and endorphins and time. Exquisite. Then I buckle it shut around his neck. What happens next depends on the boy in question, my inclination at that moment, and the mood we make together. It usually ends with him kissing my boots.

We kept meeting that way: at parties, over nibbles and sips. I overcame my initial paralysis enough to flirt back. The morning of Pink Saturday, the day before Pride Sunday, the traditional party is the brunch benefit for The Positive Resource Center. Again, I was cavorting with Christopher. We had our picture taken with Ian McKellen, who was a "celebrity" grand-marshal that year. He was charming: came to all the parties, mixed, and joked about being a "queen" of England. Alan was standing talking with a small cluster of other leathermen and since Christopher was studiously chatting up Sir Ian, I joined them.

The conversation was meandering. Who will win the annual International Mr. Leather contest? Will Gay Shame throw a couch onto the parade route again this year? Isn't the buffet quite good? Aren't Sir Ian's white linen pants amazing? They don't leave much to the imagination, do they? What about that new campaign by Stop AIDS? Is it in good taste? Or not? Who are the interesting new boys? Well, Alan still misses Johnny of course. There are lots of nice boys, but no really good contenders for special boy. There is one in Philadelphia, who could be a contender, but he lives too far away, and his business won't allow him to move. They can't see one another very often. And there is another in Sacramento who would like to be Alan's boy, but Alan is not quite feeling it. He is nice of course, and quite cute, but not quite right. But at least he's fairly local.

Finally a pause and I saw my opportunity. I took a deep breath. "Sir?" He turned towards me. "I live in Noe Valley." It was just a statement of fact. I didn't ask for anything or suggest anything. I just offered Him a piece of information . . . for Him to do with as He wished.

A cat-like small smile began to play across His lips and He tilted His head back. "Well . . . perhaps, after Pride, we could . . . meet privately."

"I would like that very much, Sir."

"Good. Then after Pride, later in the following week, call me."

"Yes, Sir."

He held my eyes for a long moment then returned to the conversation. Who is performing on the main stage? How nice that the weather is perfect for the parade tomorrow. Who is in from out of town? Who plans to run for San Francisco Leather Daddy this year? Oh, Donna Sachet is about to sing. Shall we return to our tables?

So that was it. He put it out there. I nibbled. I put it out there. He bit. But now there was a question. Not a question: THE question, the big one. Did He know about me? He might, but He might not. It might make no difference. But it might make all the difference. I had to find out. I had to at least try to find out, so I asked Peter.

"Peter . . . Daddy Alan. Does He know about me?"

"Ohhh . . . well, yes. Or . . . no. Maybe? I think so. I'm not sure. Oh, but he is very good about those kinds of things. He is very supportive. He is a great ally!"

"Ummm . . . okay. You don't know if He knows?"

"No, but I don't think it would make any difference. He is very good."

"Okay. But you know, being good politically, being a great ally is great. But it doesn't mean that you necessarily want to fuck somebody."

Peter gave me a look that suggested that this had not quite occurred to him. Peter is a great ally. Peter also gets with trans guys. No problem. I suppose it is human nature to see things through our own frames. "Ohhh . . . well. Hmmm. No. I don't know for sure whether he knows."

Now I am NOT the kind of transsexual who thinks that if someone does not want to fuck me because I am trans, that it makes him "transphobic." Desire has its own eccentric logic. It's a magical trajectory, but delicate, and it can be thrown off-course by an ill-placed "should." If someone tries too hard to get his (his? her? hir? zeer? zim's?) political and libidinal engines to sync, he can end up sexually frustrated. Or politically rotten. Or both. So . . . no. I didn't "expect" Alan to want me, and I would not have thought less of Him if He hadn't.

But I did want Him to want me. I spent the next week making inquiries. Nobody knew if He knew. I've developed a method for disclosing. It only works in San Francisco, or in other situations where I am well-known enough that there is some chance that I've been talked about in circles in my absence. I count on the fact that human beings are social animals. We like to talk to each another, and we like to talk to each other about each other. And face it. Transsexuality is a juicy dish.

Rather than be annoyed at being regularly outed, I assume that I will be and I use it. If a situation is developing that is likely to lead quickly to less clothing, I will pause and whisper as casually as possible something like: "Say . . . do you know about me?" There are really only two possible replies. One is that he will say something like: "Yes. Of course. It's okay." In which case: "Houston, we have lift-off." The other possible response is something like: "I have no idea what you are talking about." In that case, I have to tell. I don't like it, but I do it. I don't apologize. I don't explain. I don't let my voice shake or my eyes drop. I don't allow myself to betray any distaste at having to share this . . . detail. I find that the more casual I am, the more casual he will be. Usually, it's no problem. Usually, he has been assuming this was going to be the "poz" talk. If he is, this is usually when he says so, and if he is of a certain age and aesthetic mode then this is also when he shows me the biohazard tattoo. We all bear our history on and in our flesh and our marks and our scars are proof: it is up to us to bear them with honesty, courage, and honor.

I called Alan. Gulp. We made a date. Eat? No. We've nibbled plenty. But we have never been alone. Tomorrow afternoon. I'll be at the Center. He will pick me up. We will go to His place. Okay. Tomorrow. "Thank You, Sir." Click.

The next day, I met him outside of the Center. I had decided to tell Him in His truck. My thinking was: if my "T" was going to be a deal-killer, I wanted to know that right away. If it was going to be "thanks, but no thanks" then I could have Him drop me off at home and I could spend the rest of the afternoon and evening alone, licking my wounds. I'd be fine again by the next day. I had carefully not invested too much too soon.

But, oh: I did want Him and I did want Him to want me. I like men a lot and I like a lot of men. But some men, a very few, really flip my switch. However, I'm no kid and I'm not easily swept away. For it to be a go, everything has to check out. I had about ten minutes to find the right spot in the conversation.

I was a very cute boy. Very smart. Very charming. Very sexy. Alan was never stingy with compliments but as we drove He kept glancing over at me, running His eyes over me and doing what my mother would have called "laying it on thick." He turned the conversation to sex fast. Did I enjoy getting fucked? Yes? Oh, good. And, yes Sir, a very good cocksucker. Kinky? Well, of course. Bondage? Yes. Domination? Yes. A Switch: but very submissive, very good, very obedient—with only those very few men who flip that particular switch—

Sir. And I held His eyes long and hard. He smiled, seeming to like that and to like a boy who can understand his own power and who knows he is giving up something real and valuable when he turns it over.

Yes, I know hanky code. Yes, I have seen that He flags red and gray. Handball is divine . . . of course. (But His hands are Huge!) Piss is nice, but scat is messy. Well, we seem to agree on quite a bit, have tastes in common. He is not too much of a sadist. Okay. But how is it that such an amazing boy has not been scooped up? Well, I am very choosy. Of course. And I am complicated in certain ways. Not high-maintenance, just . . . unusual. I looked over to Him searching for insight, a sign that He might have read this hint, but I found none. He was quiet for a long moment.

"Complicated? Whatever do you mean?"

I inhaled deeply, but not for long. We were drawing close to His house. "Well, Sir, do you know about me?"

He turned slowly towards me, raised His eyebrows and I knew the answer. "I have no idea what you are talking about."

(Matter of fact. Casual. How's the weather? No big deal.) "Sir, I am transsexual."

He turned quickly towards me then turned back to the road. After a moment, He turned back and looked at my face, my body, my face. He shook his head, turned away, turned back, and smiled. This took ten years.

"Reeeaally! How marvelous! I had no idea!"

This was not quite what I had expected.

"You know . . . some of the best sex I have ever had was with an FTM boy from Vancouver. His name is Dennis. Do you know him I wonder?"

"No, Sir. I don't know him."

"No idea at all. How very exciting!"

We pulled into His garage. We went into His house. He sat in His chair. I knelt at His feet. He wore very soft ancient Levi's and boots. I undid His belt with my teeth, and unbuttoned His 501s with my lips. I showed Him some of my skills: a very good boy. He wore a snapping leather cock-ring. He wasn't young, but He was strong. And big! When I was a child, I used to practice holding my breath; 30 seconds, 45 seconds, one minute. On road trips, I would use the mile markers to time myself. Sixty miles an hour: I'd gulp a lungful at one marker and exhale at the next. Practicing for I didn't know what. He made us something to eat. I washed up. He told me about Johnny. And Pete.

We were together for two years. It felt natural. We knew one another. I recognized Him the first time I saw Him, years before we met. Some people are just like that. When we first got together we talked about my leaving. I was planning to go to graduate school. I was to become a doctor of philosophy. We agreed that saying yes to embarking on a relationship and having some time close by and then some time visiting made more sense than saying no because of what might or might not happen. Who knows how long any of us has and who knows how long any of us have together? The end comes quickly enough. A year in the same town; another year of visits; a priceless gift; an amazing man. He took me to the best parties, black leather and black tie, always proudly introducing me as His boy, sometimes embarrassing me by gushing about me in front of me. A big famous leatherman, a lifelong Top, He was the sweetest individual I have ever known, and probably the sweetest I will ever know.

Sometimes I would accompany Him on His rounds: collecting donations for the endless benefits. He raised maybe half a million dollars for people with AIDS during His fundraising career. And that was for direct assistance: electricity bills were paid, the gas stayed on and food came. For twenty years, He volunteered at ward 5B: holding the hands and massaging the pain-wracked bodies of the mostly young and often abandoned men who filled those beds. And feeding people at Tenderloin Tessie's on Thanksgiving: We would pull into a space in front of a bakery, and Alan would walk in smiling and cheerfully declare, "I have come for the pies!" Minutes later, I'd be loading fifty donated pies into the truck. No one could say no to Him. That was Alan.

He adored me and I adored Him. He even taught me to take Him: no mean feat. He had a phoenix tattooed on His right arm and a dragon on His left. He would joke about using the phoenix as a depth-gauge. The beak pointed to His wrist, the fiery tail feathers ran to His elbow. "When the tail feathers disappear . . . well!" This was a man who could reach into a boy and hold his beating heart in His hand. And He was always perfect with me. He made me feel cherished, and sexy. He held my heart in His hand. He told me I had a beautiful body and made me believe it. We never once said a single unkind word to one another.

Shortly before I went to Southern California to grad school, I met a kid, a young trans man: a messy teenager who was smart and strong and fierce and gorgeous. He's an androphile like me: he loves his men and he is tough. This boy became my son by affiliation. It's not a sex thing; it's a love and a family thing. That is what affiliation is at its root: "filia"—it originally meant taking on a son—not adopting an infant you don't know, but taking on a young man you do. He is twenty-three now. I am very proud of him. And Alan treated him like a grandson. It is important to take care of one another. I know that. My son Aidan knows it. Alan knew it. It is about trust and honor and respect. Genuine Leather.

Alan told me when He would go and that was when He went. At The Folsom Street Fair the previous fall He had said that this would be His last Folsom. I believed it. He had "lost his puff," as He put it in His inimitable boys' school English. He called me one day the following spring and said: "I think I will go the Sunday after the AEF Gala. I do want to go to my last Gala." He was sick. Not many people knew. I knew. A few close friends knew. He didn't want many people to know. He did not want to linger and He really did not want anyone to fuss or hover.

He wanted to go out and do things and see people and flirt with the boys. He wanted everyone to see Him as He was: cheerful and strong, and He would have been aghast at any show of sadness or pity or to be thought of as a man who was dying. He wasn't dying; He was living. He had explained to me that He planned to live life fully until very close to the end and that when He went it would be very fast. That is the way He wanted it and that is the way He did it. No fatal dose of anything: just pure force of will. How incredible . . . and how very typical of Him.

We had been sitting bedside since midnight: me and Aidan and the Daddies Tony and André and the boy Jorge. We had been there for days, on and off, a small shifting group. No one was sleeping much. It had been a week since the Gala: His last outing. He had eaten a few bites of a favorite meal of duck days before. I held Him, and whispered that He would be seeing Johnny soon and to please tell him "thank you" from me. He murmured and smiled and squeezed my hand. Every two hours, we slid morphine into the space between His gum and cheek to make His labored breathing easier. Jorge kept the hot coffee and cold washcloths coming: a very good boy.

We put His leather cap with its silver eagle ornament onto His chest and wrapped His hot dry hands around it. Early Sunday morning He gasped hard and died. I held His warm, still, quiet body. The animal part of my brain could not comprehend how His skin could be warm and soft but at the same time He didn't breathe or pulsate. Tony called Daddies Steve and Peter and the undertakers. They came. The undertakers were two deaf lesbians with impeccable manners who were garbed in something like Edwardian male drag: His favorites. Of course . . . He had buried so many of His own and He wanted these two fabulous women. Steve, Peter, André, and Tony are San Francisco Leather Daddies: numbers twelve, twenty-one, fourteen, and twenty. Alan was the original. He started the contest as a fundraiser for His beloved AEF. No number. Zero: no beginning and no end.

Daddy Peter is a great guy, a good friend, and a skillful, knowledgeable, and well-respected leatherman. He's also a big proponent of including trans leathermen in men's leather events and organizations. And almost all do. But Chicago's ancient and generally well-respected Hellfire Club had at this time just narrowly voted in a "born-male" policy. Their stance is stupid, and a lot of their members know that. Me? I support anyone's right to be a wrong-headed bigot. But Peter, who is not trans, takes any exclusion as a personal affront to his sense of fair play. A long-time Hellfire member, he resigned and stripped their distinctive "colors" from his bar vest. This left an instantly recognizable and provocatively unworn shiny spot where the patch had once been.

I suspect that Alan's death was so jarring that Peter responded by choosing this moment to launch into a Hellfire tirade. I glanced at my kid and could read the mortification in his eyes. He had just started transitioning and looked either ambiguous or thirteen. He did not know most of these men. He stared at me wordlessly, silently begging intervention. But nothing about my upbringing or the social hierarchy of the assembled group or my leather training allowed me to tell Peter to please just shut the hell up. So I looked at him blankly, hoping he would stop it and leave his well-placed and righteous annoyance for a more appropriate moment. No luck there, but then, Steve spoke. "Well, they are just wrong. Trans men are men and soon Hellfire will get that and things will change and that will be that." And that was that. There was nothing more to be said and nothing more was said. He had backed Peter up while simultaneously shutting him down.

Nobody lost face. I started to pay attention to how he handled himself: more genuine leather.

We went back to saying goodbye. Aidan pulled the collar out of Alan's bedside table and presented it to me, as he had promised Alan he would do. The other things came later, as Tony and I went through His things. I wear His belt daily. It reminds me of who and what I am. We sent Alan's body away with the fancy morticians. Tony growled at a neighbor who gawked as we followed the body to the waiting hearse and it was over. At Alan's packed celebration of life two weeks later, I delivered a short eulogy:

> Daddy Alan Selby was an Englishman who became an American. He was a gentleman and He was a leatherman. He was the original Daddy, the ultimate Daddy, the Daddy of all Daddies, and He was my Daddy. He loved me and I loved Him. I miss Him already and I will miss Him always. However, His passage was no tragedy. He lived His life with good humor, courage, compassion, generosity and grace. If we can incorporate these characteristics, apply them to our lives and impart them to the generations coming up, then the spirit of this great man will never die. I would like to say, then, in the words of His countryman, not "good bye" but "good night, sweet Daddy. (Jordy Jones, at the SF Eagle, May 23, 2004)

21

Love Lost and Found

Martine Delaney

Most mornings of my life, I'm dragged from slumber by the sound of one tail wagging: Saffy, the larger of our mixed-breed bed-warmers. She of the need for fixed routine, believes 6:00 a.m. is toilet time; for her, if not for me. She stands patiently by the bed, wagging her tail to wake me. And so begins another day with feeding her and Jake, the Jack Russell "Terrorist," filling bowls for the seven cats, and preparing breakfast for my partner and I. On workdays, I make lunch to go.

It's all incredibly mundane, perhaps even potentially boring. But, it seldom seems so to me. I rise and feed the beasts each day, make meals and break the fast in a blissful and probably annoyingly bubbly manner. Because I'm in love and I am loved; it's as simple as that, and a totally unexpected place for me to be.

In matters of love, I believe myself to have been blessed—far more than I deserve or could, in any way, expect. In both guises by which my world has known me, I've been gifted with love of an extraordinary nature; twice sharing my life in relationships most people hope for, but seldom find. At least, that's how it seems to me and I'm smugly comfortable with the idea.

In telling you of my life and love as a trans person, I see no way of doing justice to my tale without telling also of my life and love as a closeted trans person. That earlier life, its unfolding and its dark moments, forever influences the manner in which I live my days and share them with my love. Author Douglas Adams' creation, Dirk Gently, the holistic investigator, solves mysteries by studying the interconnectedness of all things in the universe; how the fluttering of a butterfly's wings, on a fictitious distant planet, influences events here on earth. My lives and loves, then and now, tell me he speaks the truth.

I'm a trans woman. It would be wonderful to be able to tell of my extraordinary journey to the making of that simple statement. And, for me, it has often seemed an extraordinary time. However, from hearing the stories of others and armed now with hindsight, it's really been about as ordinary as my morning routine. We all travel different paths, and some have taken their own roads to arrive at a place much like mine, but we are all subject to the demands and expectations of the world around us, to forces which shape us, leading to as many similarities in our singular, extraordinary journeys as there might be differences. I've no doubt many others could tell my tale as their own.

I was born the fourth of seven children—the fourth of five successive males—into a solid, working-class, Catholic family in Tasmania, Australia. As far back as I remember, my mother was crippled by a spinal condition, hospitalized for months at a time and usually recuperating from surgery. Our home, then, was a macho place—dominated by its maleness with football, cricket, and being a boy the usual business of the day. And by the age of five, in this house of men, I knew I was supposed to be a girl. No clear justification for the proposition, nor understanding why, but an amazing conviction that has stayed with me ever since, one which set my course for the next twenty-five years.

Not family, school, nor my community offered encouragement to the notion of gender transitioning as a career choice. So, I devoted myself to proving to the world—and myself—just how much of a boy I really was. Class clown, troublemaker, teenage drinker, and girl-chaser, I played them all. By my late teens, life was all about serious team sports, alcohol, and powerful cars. Without doubt, I was a *bona fide* lad. A lad who spent much of her time daydreaming of clothes, names, and her life as a woman.

Barely twenty-two years of age, I married. To a woman whose greatest fault was wanting all those things I needed as proof of my normalcy: a suburban house, a middle-class collection of antiques, travel, a social life, and successful careers. Sadly, I can't speak of this marriage in any discussion of my loves. I was incredibly fond of her and she loved me dearly or, at least the image of me I was so keen to show the world. It wasn't love that led me to marry, but the shelter given by the pretence. Today, I can only feel disappointed with my-self for my dishonesty and abuse of her love, along with anger at my birth into a society where such dishonesty seemed a reasonable choice to make, an acceptable response to the problem of being different.

By thirty, I'd devoted a couple of years to destroying my wife's love. Still unable to be honest, I planned to drive her from me and flee to the Monash Gender Clinic, my life and transition bankrolled by my share of the sale of our middle-class life. My plan was working, the ship of our marriage broken on the rocks, when I rather complicated proceedings. I fell in love, deeply in love, for the first time in my life.

I'd spent years working in the social justice field and she was a col-league, widowed, a mother to two young boys. Her presence, our con-versations, our silences, lit up my life so amazingly. And confused me, derailed me, placed huge obstacles in the smooth path of my plans. To add to my problems, she then confessed her love for me. Obviously, I had a decision to make—run for my life or be painfully truthful about who and what I was. I knew I couldn't be part of an-other relationship founded on my dishonesty, but the notion of expos-ing my secret was utterly terrifying, almost debilitating. In the end, I opted for honesty.

She was in love, heterosexual, and devastated by my news. In her own words, she thought she'd finally found her knight in shining ar-mor—and I wanted to be her princess! The idea of a same-sex rela-tionship, with a woman who'd been her boyfriend, did nothing for her. We were both perturbed by the thought of introducing me to her sons as a new father figure who'd one day become a second mum! In the end, though, love prevailed. After months of deep discussion, we settled on a plan—life as a straight couple until the boys were inde-pendent; they'd not had easy childhoods and we wanted to give them some stable time. Then, we'd try our same-sex relationship. With a proviso; she felt some guilt at the postponement of my plans and ex-tracted from me a promise that I'd go ahead with my move to woman-hood if anything should happen to her. I gave the promise freely, madly in love and knowing our life would last forever. For the first time ever, I was sharing my truth with another.

Finally, somewhat long-windedly, I've brought you to the first of my loves. It's not the love I sat down to write about. In many ways, it has no place in a collection of the lives and loves of trans people. Except, in its genesis and ending, it has a great bearing on the trans woman I've become and the way in which I love today.

Firstly, importantly, it began with an honesty I'd never shared before. It grew and flourished. We moved this wonderful, honest love to the home we built, half-built, in a hillside paddock looking out across a lagoon painted daily by swirling, orange sunrises. The house was still half-built when I sold it twelve years later—the victim of too many conversations, people to share life with, animals to care for, and an unexpected ending. Our horse and donkeys kept the paddock trim and our home was filled with our boys, their friends, cats, dogs, and a constant stream of children needing refuge from a harsh world. I would think of something incredibly important to tell her, and she'd speak it as I formed the words. She'd phone to remind me to buy hay for the donkeys; I'd be slow to answer because I was struggling to get an extra bale in the back of the station wagon. Shared anger at society's inequities inspired our work and led to conversations lasting into the early hours, to be rekindled in the morning over coffee on the sun-drenched deck; interrupted by the need to decide on arriving at work just an hour late, or making more coffee and talking some more of today's important things.

As the years passed, we began to speak more often of my future. Our older boy had returned from two years of backpacking through Europe with his girlfriend and they'd taken up residence in their own wee nest. Our younger was on his first flatting adventure with a friend. We were sharing our home with a young girl who needed shelter after a nine-year life of neglect, abuse, and abandonment. But, there was space to consider the very scary prospect of whether our love could survive my journey. We talked and we worried, and we steeled ourselves for that future. Then, she was gone, and I'd not steeled myself for that.

We'd talked and sipped coffee in the morning light. Joked and kissed sweetly before I left to finish preparations for a festival I was managing. On holidays from work, she was taking our fosterling and a friend to walk the dogs at her favorite beach. There, that day—our plans, my life, our love—went badly awry. It seems she spent some thirty minutes rescuing one of the children from an undertow. Just moments later, exhausted, she was knocked off her feet by a wave, unable to rescue herself. The sea, oh-so-thoughtfully, returned her body to the children a half-hour later.

She was gone and I was not, but I was—in many, many ways. I grieved, as I do to this day. In the months after, I spread her ashes at the beach, took back responsibility for our foster child, returned to work and walked through life, disconnected. Eventually, I kept my promise and began to explore the process of gender reassignment. A year after her death, I was on hormones and the path to my own brand of womanhood; still grieving, aware I could never know if our life would have survived that road.

So, as I mentioned, I'm a trans woman. One very much shaped by my life and that love, which leads me to yet more digression from the life and love I'm supposedly writing of. No differently to all others in this world, I make choices and must live with the consequences of those choices. Implicit in this right to choose is the notion that others have an equal right to choose differently than myself. Ergo, I've friends and acquaintances who were once trans folk. They transitioned, underwent surgery in most cases, and no longer see themselves as trans folk—just men and women living their lives in a world which seldom, if ever, notices them. I respect their choices and admire their courage. Such choices bring their own consequences, different than mine but no less worrying and ever present.

Had I been born into a different world, one more celebratory and accepting of difference, I might also have chosen to fly stealth through the gender skies. I have often wished I could pass through life as just another woman, treated no differently, no better or worse, than other women. But, I wasn't born into that world and so I've chosen to embrace, even promote, my previous life as a part of me. And, I doubt I could ever afford the surgery I'd need to hide the evidence of more than forty years of testosterone-fed life. Besides, it's just the most amazing fun to watch the faces of your former classmates when you arrive at the thirty-year reunion dinner of a Catholic, boys-only school!

Let's try again, with feeling and determination . . . I am a trans woman. To assist those who are aided by labels, I'm transsexual, male-to-female, post-op and autogynephilic—the latter according to Canadian sexologist Ray Blanchard, trans doctor Anne Lawrence, and author J. Michael Bailey. I see myself simply as me, and I find the labels somewhat limiting, often divisive, and inevitably demeaning to someone. So, I am just me, simply me, no more nor less than the sum of all that has made my life to date. Which means I am very much shaped by that earlier, aforementioned life and love. Having found in-credible happiness in that love—within the only relationship I'd com-menced with total honesty—I now see such honesty as essential to living my life. I cannot envisage presenting myself to the world in a less-than-honest manner, as anything other than "*moi*" in all my flawed glory.

Where once I felt the need for a wardrobe full of faces and per-sonae to suit each occasion, I now dress myself as the same me for the whole world; swap the accessories, perhaps to suit the particular rela-tionship—partner, lover, foster-care giver, step-parent, friend—as each requires a different brooch or bag, but the basic outfit remains very much the same.

So, I pass by not passing. I present my past as my past; and if that doesn't pass, then I pass—because I'm past it! Which is all, actually, so very easy. I don't need to tiptoe through my world, remember any-thing but my real life story, or ever worry about my voice giving me away. It can never give me away; rather, it advertises my presence, my reality and my difference. And, my reality and difference have a pur-pose. Each time a call-center worker is forced to consider whether she can discuss Ms. Delaney's insurance policy with a masculine-voiced me, or the sales assistant needs to think about how to address me, my difference has a purpose—it forces others to ponder the concept of di-versity and, perhaps, to begin considering all difference as normal.

By remaining true to the honesty born of my lost love, I am able to use me as a small tool for social change in my little corner of the world—a vanilla-oiled, sandalwood-scented, oestrogen-enhanced slap in the face to those who've not yet noticed, accepted, and cele-brated diversity. It's not my raison d'être, but it gives me additional purpose and certainly keeps boredom at bay! I can be ok with the ri-diculous tabloid headline of "Sex-change Soccer Star," if my pres-ence in a women's soccer team causes even a few to think about the issues. Maybe, some day, this might lead to nobody seeing gender di-versity as an issue requiring thought?

While that lost love gave much direction to my life beyond, it also meant the end of love. Having loved as deeply, as sweetly, as we had loved, I knew that part of my life was gone. I could not, and did not, consider I would ever love again—or believe any attempt to love might be granted fair chance in comparison with those lost times. I wasn't the slightest bit worried at such a thought, I just didn't believe I could ever love again.

While not seeking or believing in future love I also found I'd become asexual. To this day, I've no idea whether this was as a result of my long-lived grief, my breakfasts of oestrogen and anti-androgens, or a combination of both. It certainly didn't worry me; since I'd never love again, asexuality was quite a comfortable state of being and, for a couple of years, I was an uncomplaining resident of that state. I stayed there contentedly until the night Adonis strolled into a Hobart pub and did some damage to my understanding of myself.

In my other life, I had always been a happily heterosexual male—while wishing since childhood to have a female body of my own, I'd still found the female form attractive and desirable. Some men I'd see as good-looking, but I was never attracted to them. I assumed, as a trans woman, I'd continue to find women attractive—if ever I emerged from my cocoon of asexuality. Adonis, however, forced me to reconsider. Heading home to Olympus, he popped into the pub to share a beer with friends while I was sharing a bottle of bubbly with a girlfriend.

We shared nothing, Adonis and I, and I'm sure he didn't notice us at all. I, however, noticed several new things while staring at his beauty. My stomach became empty, hollowed out, and full of the strangest sensations. My legs grew weak and wobbly; and, for at least a minute, I was unable to close my gaping mouth! Having never experienced such a reaction as a man towards either girls or boys, I decided I must have arrived as a straight female. Nothing came of it—he disappeared with friends, while I sat stupidly on a stool until my legs began to function again. But I was a little clearer about what I was: a healthy, straight, out-there trans girl with almost no expectations of my life changing too much from there.

A few other things happened along the way. Having truly fled the confines of the closet, and with a long involvement in social justice issues, I soon found myself on the management committee of Working It Out, a support service for lesbian, gay, bisexual, and transgender Tasmanians. I looked death in the eye and chatted with the Grim Reaper while having two heart attacks. Underwent reassignment surgery, recuperated, returned to my work and found myself retrenched. I should have expected it, since my boss had ceased speaking to me directly, preferring e-mail as an alternative, shortly after my boobs had grown larger than her own. Two weeks after getting back to work, I was out of work. Forced to sell my half-built house, because the mortgage was a whole lot more than the government offered as a salary replacement. I also became an unsuspecting victim of love!

During my first Working It Out committee meeting, I was one of four new members of the board, all the fruit of a successful recruiting drive to boost falling numbers. One of the other newbies, JP, really annoyed me. Small guy, very slightly camp, hairy neck, and the George Michael look, badly in need of a shave. He kept poking his nose into transgender issues, offering opinions and taking on tasks— a veritable little gay tranny-hag! After a month and another meeting, I was close to hitting him, so annoyed was I by his condescending gay man's interference in trans issues. Thought about it some more, slapped my own face and the light came on—he was a trans man!

Talked to him about that and confirmed my initial stupidity. We became friends, spending quite a lot of our free time together, along with his then-partner and Jenna, another of the new committee members. Despite being trans all my life, the issues and politics were new to me and I was loving it. On occasions when I was fosterling-free and Jenna wasn't busy with her boyfriend, we'd go clubbing and I'd explore my newfound status as a girl in the world—eyeing off the boys, left feeling powerless and weak by a leather-clad woman who took me where she wanted on the dance floor, when she wanted, and asked not my views. Jenna thought that was really quite funny!

Love made its sneak attack while Jenna was on holidays for a family wedding, the justification for her to spend three weeks away on the mainland. Not too long after she'd left, I was phoning her several times a day and feeling totally bereft, lost, on days I was unable to speak to her. I didn't actually admit any of this until a few days after her return, at a mutual friend's birthday gathering. While people danced and partied around us, I spent most of the night attempting to tell Jenna I'd fallen in love with her. She sat there, smiling at me, letting me stumble through my explanation, smiling and not making it at all easy. Smiling because, as she eventually shared with me, she felt the same way about me.

I know we met at that first management committee meeting and I sat next to her at a dinner afterwards. But I'd barely spoken to her at either event, and my memory of her from that day consists more, in hindsight, of guilt and sadness at ignoring her presence than it does of a memory of her presence. For me, we met over a period of months, our friendship grew in the following year and then we became lovers overnight.

Jenna is my love, my light, and my inspiration. For some years, I had walked through life detached from those around me; interested and, in some ways, inspired by the changes in me and the world opening up before me but, on a personal level, feeling little and with no joy in my life and heart. That changed with Jenna. Simply by being Jenna, she brought life to my soul, light to my world and meaning to my life. Over time, without me noticing, she had rekindled a spark extinguished by a big wave on a deserted beach some years before.

Where I talked with others and enjoyed the conversation, with Jenna the conversations flew, brought new ideas and directions, inspired me in ways I'd long forgotten. She has the most amazing way of knowing how others feel, of empathizing with all people, of leading me to see something of the place in which others live and of how they view the world. She can share my anger at injustice, but temper the response by perceiving ways in which those things might have come to pass. We suspect it might be the purpose of her journey in this life, to achieve balance by experiencing both sides of all situations, by seeing each side of every coin. Along with inspiration, she has brought balance to my life.

This latter aspect of my Jenna is clearly evidenced by her journey to bisexuality. She arrived in Tasmania, some years ago, a straight woman in a straight relationship; discovered same-sex attraction and had a couple of girlfriends and a boyfriend. In true Jenna fashion, she seemed to take not very long to deduce it was the individual she was attracted to—not gender or genitalia—and attractive, sexy people weren't found just among the opposite sex.

Not only is my Jenna entirely comfortable with her sexuality, bringing me to clarity on my own bisexuality, she is also incredibly at home with public displays of our relationship. Where I began with fear, noticing every pointed finger, hearing every whispered comment about my appearance or our hand-holding, she simply refused to notice, to accept such attitudes could exist in a just world. So, they didn't, and she has brought me to understand that such prejudice can only harm if I give it breath by accepting it. Her strength of belief in the rightness of who we are has made me so much stronger, so much more than I was and so much more in love with her.

Should I ever tire of loving Jenna for her nature and mind, I could happily spend eternity drowning in the depths of her amazingly dark, brown, and beautiful eyes; fill myself with joy, gazing upon her sleeping form, her face so gorgeous and serene at rest; stare in awe at her upon the dance floor, lost to me as the beat takes her to other spaces—her hips, her arms, all of her, moving in ways I could never hope to emulate; or simply wallow in the sensation of heat and dizziness she can create in me with her touch, with a kiss.

I'm not sure why she fell in love with me. She's explained it a few times: things to do with my sense of humor, intellect, my passion for justice, love of animals, and the fact I enjoy cooking and usually manage to produce tasty meals. Surprisingly, to me, she seems to also find me attractive. But the reasons matter not at all—I know I am loved, and I love her dearly. My being with Jenna allows me to nurture, to share, and to grow with so little apparent effort. In return, I find myself supported, inspired and cared for, loved completely for who I am, despite my dainty feet of clay. When I doubt myself, I know Jenna believes in me and the campaigning work I do—often having, I suspect—more faith in me than I have in myself. But, it is a beautiful, truly beautiful, relationship to be sharing, and I can only thank the Goddess daily for my fortune. Having once been certain I'd not find love again, I now know myself to have been twice blessed by this universe.

Sound idyllic? It's wonderful, and I shall never cease to thank the gods, goddesses, the universe—whoever, whatever—responsible for my fortune. But it wasn't easy to reach this point, nor is it easy to remain here. And, I must take responsibility for much of that. As written earlier, I am shaped by my other life and love; while these created in me a strong and proud trans woman, they also planted seeds of doubt—doubt of my worth and ability to be part of this relationship, and doubts about its future.

Fortunately, we survived the first of the difficulties I brought to our relationship. A penis—or, more correctly, a lack of a penis. No matter how much of my life I daydreamed about its disappearance, of a life without it, that penis had been with me in every relationship I'd known. And, the damn thing shaped me, and my relationships, on all levels. No matter how hard you try, with one of those in your knickers there's always an element of "man" involved in getting to know someone. With Jenna, I entered my first ever penis-free relationship and I had not a clue! I was where I'd wanted to be for such a long time, and I'd no idea where to go now that I'd gotten there. But Jenna, my gentle Jenna, she showed me the ways; she led me to places I'd never known, emotionally and physically, and brought me to believe I belonged. She is truly beautiful and I thank her, for all time, for her knowing of the ways.

Still, Jenna came to our relationship with doubts. She'd loved before, committed herself completely to others who spoke of their undying love; who continued to speak of their undying love, until its death was marked by their departure. So, cynicism had become a part of her outlook on life and love. I'm sure she's now convinced my love for her is, indeed, undying, and of my commitment to her for all time. Though I worry I may have inflicted upon her my other fears for our life together.

From the moment I acknowledged my love for Jenna, I've been certain this love would last forever; and, just as certain she will love me for all time. I do not doubt, at all, the strength of our love and relationship. Yet, each day, I fear for them. For I had loved before, certain it would be for all time, and then had my love torn from me by a wave and tossed back, lifeless, on the shore. I know the certainty of love, however great that love might be, cannot reach beyond the uncertainty of life.

As if to add to this lesson from my other life and love, the universe provided a reminder, a truly cruel reminder, just days ago. We'd risen early, walked the dogs in the crisp dawn air, shared a leisurely breakfast. Up early, we returned to bed to read for a while before work. Between us on the duvet, our two youngest cats gave us the pleasure of their company. Their mother—tiny, thin, and pregnant—had adopted us some months before. She gave birth to four amazing kittens in an antique cauldron in our hallway. Jenna witnessed the birthing, her first such experience. Dave, the last-born, was fortunate she was there—weak and tiny, he seemed destined to die; she spent several hours coaxing him to feed, warming him and putting him on the teat until he'd worked the system out.

Dave, his mother, and one brother had remained with us. He had grown from runt to exquisite young man. Solid and muscular, a small ginger-on-ginger tiger cub; placid, golden eyes gazing on me as he purred, he seemed to enjoy our reading time as much as we did. At five months, he gave glimpses of the beautiful creature he would become.

A very short time later—as I sat here to write of my fears for our love—our trusting, gorgeous Dave wandered into a neighbor's yard and was killed in seconds by their dog, his body crushed and made lifeless by powerful, ugly, slobbering, stupid jaws. And there's the rub, really; the other part of my earlier life shaping my love today. You can, like Dave, love and trust completely, expecting it all to go on forever; you can love unconditionally, as we did and we now do, knowing it is forever. But it really doesn't matter, because there is no guarantee you'll have the opportunity to express that love tomorrow—no matter how strong, how great your loving.

And thus my love is shaped. I never doubt its strength and beauty, but I constantly fear its sudden disappearance, its passing without me having shared it enough. So, I've made the expression of love second nature to my day; perhaps this drives Jenna crazy, but she's not asked me to stop so I continue to tell her of my love all day—never leaving a room without an "I love you" and a kiss, never wishing the sun to set or me to sleep with bad feelings unresolved. In return, she shows her true beauty in her acceptance of my fears, her ever-present love for me despite the frequent tears for lives and loves lost long ago.

It has survived much, this love, besides my fears and foibles. Saffydog—who needed to sit between us and separate our hands—until the day she realized I was someone who would also feed her regularly and she learned to love me for that. My fosterling, who found it almost impossible to share me and chose eventually to live her life elsewhere; my mother, who seemed certain I would find a nice man and settle down in suburbia. My siblings, who genuinely seem fond of Jenna but struggle with all concepts beyond "straight couple with kids." And, finally, all those people who whisper, point, and stare—sad people, Jenna has taught me, who have no meaning in our world if we don't give it. It survives all these things, grows each day and will continue to do so for as long as the universe grants us our time for loving.

It is sad, though, to know we live and love so beautifully in a country where we are treated as second-class citizens. While our Island State places our relationship on an equal footing with married and straight de-facto couples for purposes of state-based law, nationally we just don't exist in the blind eyes of the law—except in regard to some terrorism legislation! Our loves and lives are labeled threats to the bedrock structures of society, too dangerous for recognition. It's truly sad to think people who believe themselves capable of governing our land cannot distinguish between love and weapons of mass destruction.

22

From Queer to Eternity

Zayne Jones

Giving birth to my daughter in May of 1995 inspired me to wonder what I believed my life could become. After some in-depth soul searching I realized I was extremely attracted to women. This is not to say that I hadn't been in love with my daughter's father. I just knew that being with him was not right for me. I realized that if there was one thing I wanted to teach my daughter it was that you are responsible for your own happiness. Additionally, that no one should look to someone else to complete him or her or to make him or her happy. At the end of the day I had to discover what made me feel happy with myself to set a good example.

In January of 1996 I came out as a lesbian. I was twenty-three years old and was attracted to women, so I thought that this was who I was. I believed at that time I was a lesbian. As time went by I dated women and had a couple of long-term relationships. I soon recognized that I perceived my feelings and experiences from a male gendered perspective not a female perspective. I started doing some research into the idea that it could be possible to feel male on the inside even though all my life I had been seen as female.

It was at this point in my life that one of my very close friends introduced me to a friend of hers who is FTM. Over the course of the next year he and I became very close. Through meeting him I realized all I read in books could actually happen to me if I decided that I wanted to transition. I found myself completely consumed by the idea of transitioning. I couldn't wait to start the process. However, I had to think about how this would affect my daughter who at this point was

Trans People In Love

seven years old. I definitely didn't want to disrupt or harm the relationship she and I had. I was hungry for as much information about the transition process that I could find. I looked to the Internet and many books to cure my cravings. Over the next year it became clear to me that my life as Krista was coming to a close and I just needed to figure out how to bring my life as Zayne into existence.

I started by telling my close friends whom I considered family. They all accepted me with open arms. The only exception was my girlfriend at the time. She made it clear to me that she wanted to be with a girl. Since I was no longer considering myself female she and I decided to part ways. This is when the love of my life walked in like a warm ray of sunshine and took hold of me. The woman I am speaking of goes by the name Tami. I had known Tami for about six years but we were not really friends, more like acquaintances at this point.

The first time I met Tami it was the summer of 2000. My girlfriend and I had gone to the City Diner where Tami was our waitress. You could tell just by looking at her that she was a lesbian so I decided to ask her about the gay/lesbian scene since my girlfriend and I had just moved to St. Louis from Sacramento. Throughout the next four years I ran into Tami at the bars, the Diner, and Mokabe's, the local lesbian-owned coffee house. By this time I had broken up with my girlfriend and was in an open relationship with a girl I had been seeing for three years.

In November 2004 I was at Mokabe's reading when Tami came in with one of her friends. They sat down at my table because the place was so crowded. They started telling me about Tami's bad day—she had been dumped and was ready to go out to the bars and celebrate being single once again. They invited me to come along and at first I hesitated but I soon found out that Tami doesn't take no very easily, so I gave in. A few hours later we were all headed out to Novaks, the best lesbian bar in town. As the night went on we were all drinking and having a good time, and Tami and I were getting pretty comfortable with each other. At one point I started to talk to a friend of mine, who is also FTM, and when I was done, Tami asked what we were talking about. I told her that my friend was FTM and that I was thinking of transitioning as well. We didn't really get into specifics, after all it was Friday night, but she understood what I meant by wanting to transition.

One of the things she told me, after I asked if she would ever date someone who was FTM even though she considers herself a lesbian was that she considers sexuality to be fluid and always changing. She said she doesn't think anyone should limit himself or herself when it comes to love or attraction. We spent all night talking and getting to know each other better. At the end of the night I didn't want to go home, I wanted to stay with Tami. I felt so incredibly comfortable with her. After everything I told her I never felt like she was judging me. That in itself was a wonderful feeling.

The next morning I couldn't wait to see Tami, but I couldn't decide whether or not to call. Was it too early? Does she want to see me? I decided to take my chances and call her up and see if she wanted to get coffee. Tami told me a couple of months later that she was so excited to see me again that she rushed so fast to meet up with me that she forgot to put on deodorant. We spent all day talking and learning about each other, and the more I learned about her the more I realized she was someone I could really fall in love with.

Over the next two weeks we spent all of our free time together and Tami was even able to meet my nine-year-old daughter. They hit it off beautifully. I knew things between them would be good when I had to leave for a few hours and my daughter wanted to stay with Tami instead of leaving with me. When I got back from my errand, my daughter was asleep on Tami's lap. For me this was perfect; I had finally met someone who accepted me for me and she loves my daughter.

By January 2005 we were living together and my daughter was calling her "mom," something she had never done with anyone I had dated before. It was very out of the blue; we were putting her to bed and she just asked Tami if it would be ok if she called her mom. Tami almost cried, and of course she told her yes. Things were going really well in our relationship but I knew I couldn't stay in St. Louis. I needed to go back to Sacramento. I needed to tell my family about my transition in person. I also wanted to be close to my family when I transitioned. St. Louis was nice but it wasn't my home. I also knew that St. Louis was Tami's home; it was where her friends were and where her brother was buried. I didn't think she would move just for me, especially since we had only been together for a few months. I was wrong.

I brought up the idea of moving to California one afternoon just to gauge her reaction and she didn't even think about it she just said, "Let's go." A few weeks later we had a moving sale and sold off everything we didn't need. The night before we left for California our friends threw us a little going-away party. It was a really hard night for Tami; she had a wonderful family of friends that she was leaving behind. They were a little worried about her moving so far away but they also knew that she had her mind made up. We were all set to leave. However, I still needed to tell my mom. We are extremely close, and I couldn't tell her something this big over the phone. I decided to wait and tell her in person after we got there.

In March of 2005 we packed up the moving van and headed off to Sacramento. We decided to move in with my mother who welcomed us with open arms. Moving to Sacramento was a fairly stressful time for both of us; not only was I nervous about telling my mom, but Tami hadn't even met her before we moved in with her. The only issue was that I had not told my mother that I was going to transition. When we first got to Sacramento Tami refused to call me Zayne until I told my mom. It was a little weird hearing her call me Krista, but it did encourage me to tell my mom a little bit sooner. I knew I had to tell her now.

This was a big risk, but I was ninety-nine percent sure that my mom would be supportive of me. A few days after we moved to Sacramento I decided that I would talk to my mother. I wasn't worried at all that she would ask us to leave. I had quite the opposite feeling. I knew that she would require an adjustment period, but I knew even if she didn't understand that she would accept and love me regardless. I pressed on and the conversation with my mom went just as I suspected it would.

She listened to me with full attention, as she ingested all that I had to tell her. Mom seemed to have taken the news in her stride. I know it was hard for her to wrap her mind around the gravity of everything I was telling her but she is a great woman. She accepts me for who I am even if she doesn't fully understand what I'm doing. I can't even imagine how she must have felt. Here is her daughter who once married, gave birth to a child, came out as a lesbian and was sitting before her telling her she wanted to be a he and was going to start the transition as soon as possible.

Later, my mother told me that she may not understand why I want to transition, but she loves me, is very proud of me and will always support whatever makes me happy. All my life I knew my mother would always be there to support me but I never imagined she could be so strong and truly hold up everything she has ever told me she would do for me. In September 2005 my mother helped to finance my top surgery. She also went with me to San Francisco for my pre-op appointments. Throughout my entire life I can't think of one time that my mother has not supported me.

After Tami and I moved to Sacramento and I had told my mom, I called my dad to let him know I wanted to see him so we could talk. Tami and I went to his house and proceeded to tell him about my transition. My dad told me that he thought I was going to tell him something like that. I wondered how he would have any idea. To this day I really don't know how he might have had any inclination of what I was about to tell him. In the beginning, I didn't expect him to get the name change every time or use the correct pronouns one hundred percent of the time. I just wanted him to make an effort.

At first it was a very rocky start with my dad. He told me he didn't think he was going to be able to get used to using the male pronouns but he would make an effort to use Zayne. This hurt me but I had the feeling that he would react this way. Needless to say I wasn't very optimistic about my dad's acceptance or understanding when it came to my transition. However, this wasn't a breaking point for me. I was pressing on with my transition.

In November, two weeks before I was to have surgery, my dad was trying to be supportive by letting me know if I needed someone besides Tami to take me and stay in San Francisco or if I needed money, to just let him know and he would be glad to help out in any way. Over the last year and a half I have had up and down times with my dad but this is really no different than our relationship was before my transition. To my surprise he has been doing well with the name change and he tries to remember to use correct pronouns.

I was not worried about my sister supporting me because I had previously told her in December of 2004 when she came out to St. Louis to visit us right after the Christmas holiday with my nephew. She took the news very well. My sister is my best friend, and she continues to be one of my biggest supporters. My sister has played a key role in helping talk with my parents to help them understand the transition process, which I was about to embark on.

About three months after we moved to Sacramento I officially started my transition. I mean, I had my name picked, I told my family and I got a counselor, but now I was going to see a doctor at a clinic in San Francisco to start hormone therapy. I had my first shot of testosterone on August 17, 2005. Tami was with me at all my appointments. She learned to give me my hormone shots so she could feel more like a part of the transition. For the first month Tami gave me the shot each week. Some time after the fourth or fifth shot she wasn't able to continue. I tried explaining to her that it didn't hurt, but in her mind she had convinced herself she was causing me extreme pain. She decided to stop giving me the shots. From then on I began giving the shot to myself.

Around this same time I put out a letter to all the staff and doctors that I worked with about my transition. I let everyone know that I had changed my name and would prefer them to use male pronouns; I also told them that I had started taking testosterone. I made it clear to everyone that I was open to any questions or concerns that they might have. Ever since that letter everyone has been very supportive. I haven't received any negative feedback and I feel very lucky. I really think the letter and my willingness to be open with my co-workers helped stop any gossip. I think because I work in the hospital emergency room my co-workers are more open minded than most.

While my work environment was comfortable and nonthreatening, my personal life was being torn apart. In July 2005, Tami and I sat down with my ex-husband, the father of my daughter, and told him about my transition. We thought he had taken it fairly well; he said we would work it all out and that our daughter should be everyone's first priority. We agreed. Then two weeks later we were served court papers. He was going after full custody, wanting me to only have supervised visitation in St. Louis. To make things worse, the night before we were served the papers Tami found out that I was talking to an ex-girlfriend behind her back, even though Tami had asked me not to speak to her anymore. Tami felt that this person caused too much trouble in our relationship. However, we both agreed that this would be put on the back burner for the time being so that we could put our energy into the custody battle.

I don't want to get into any specifics about the court case but I will say that it was the most stressful time in our lives. The custody case took a year and a half to settle. Thank goodness it ended well. We kept our visitation and my ex was left without a leg to stand on. During that year and a half our relationship suffered a lot. I was very focused on the court case and my transition. I had chest surgery, a bilateral mastectomy with nipple reconstruction, in November of 2005 and it made a huge difference in the way that I saw myself. Later that year I went on a men-seeking-men Web site and put up a profile. Needless to say, the communication between Tami and I was not very good at this point. She was still very angry and hurt over me lying to her about talking to my ex-girlfriend and I was afraid to talk to her about what was going on in my head. I thought she would leave me if I told her that I thought I was attracted to men. Well Tami found my profile on this Web site and couldn't believe that I would lie to her again and keep something this big from her. But again, we put all of this aside to focus on the custody case. It would be six more months until we started fixing our problems.

Putting our relationship on the back burner was not the brightest idea we have ever had. I think we were hoping that if we ignored the problems they would just go away. They didn't. It took me almost a year to fully extract myself from the ex-girlfriend, and even longer to earn Tami's trust back. The Web site was easier. I took myself off of it as soon as Tami found it and we talked about my feelings and I felt better after I knew it was ok to talk to her about it. It took a while but we managed to work through it and now we are stronger because of it. There are two things I learned about Tami: One, she loves me as much as says she does, since she is willing to put up with everything I've done, and two, she is all knowing. She finds out everything.

Neither of us was really prepared for all the changes and stress that the transition would cause. Sometimes I would forget that the transition affects Tami as much as it affects me. When I first started the transition Tami went on a bunch of Web sites to talk to significant others of trans folk. She hadn't really known any other trans people until she met me so she wanted to find out as much information as she could about the process. However, she didn't stay on the sites for very long because they only made her paranoid. Every time someone would tell her about their situation she would automatically think that whatever that FTM was going through I would go through also. For instance, if a woman told her that her FTM partner was becoming short-tempered and aggressive because of the testosterone, Tami would worry that it would be the same for me. Once she stopped visiting the Web sites she was easier to deal with. Tami has dealt with the transition one day at a time. If I was being selfish or mean she called me on it and brought me back down to earth. We now know that our relationship works much better with open communication. Tami and

I have learned to tackle our problems together with trust and honesty. Many of the issues we have gone through so far have built strong bonds in our relationship.

Tami had a hard time when we first moved to Sacramento because she wasn't sure if she wanted to be a part of the lesbian community anymore. Before we moved, a few people in St. Louis made comments to her about "taking the easy way out." They accused her of trying to "fake being straight." She was worried that we would run into that kind of thing again. But we had concerns about not being a part of the LGBT community; we both actually thought it would be a lie to ignore that part of our lives. After all, she identifies as a lesbian and I am trans; we belong in that community. But belonging to something isn't the same as fitting in. We were both very happy to find the Sacramento Gender Association. They have dinners every few weeks and through this wonderful group we were able to meet some very good people. Tami and I finally found a place where we felt comfortable.

Tami and I have had quite a few conversations about how we classify or label our relationship. We have decided that we see our relationship as a queer relationship. This is to mean not straight or gay/lesbian. Defining our relationship in these terms makes sense to us because we knew when I started my transition we would no longer fit in with the lesbian community. This is not to say that we don't go to the gay/lesbian bars or have any gay/lesbian friends. We still have all the same friends, plus new friends from all different social classes and communities of society.

Tami and I are not concerned with labels or how others see us. Our most important goal is that we know who we are as individuals and as a couple. This, we believe, will make us strong together. As Tami and I grow old together our ideas about the relationship may change but we are both certain that we will never reach the conclusion that we are a heterosexual couple. I don't feel that I would ever consider myself to be a straight man, Tami doesn't see me as one either. Our relationship is very special. All transgendered relationships are special. Tami and I have found new levels of intimacy, levels that can't be reached by hetero couples. The transition process has stripped both of us down and shown us at our most vulnerable and we still accepted each other. Without the transition we may never have gotten the chance to see each other in that light.

My past experiences and changes will always be with me. There are many FTMs who transition and go on with their lives as if being transgender is not a part of them. I embrace it. I would one day hope that my life choices have made an impact or impression on someone who needed it along their own life journey. I would ultimately like to have the chance to help others who struggle with gender issues.

As we move towards our future there are a few more issues I have to take care of. This year I will legally change my gender and name through the court system. This will legally seal my original birth certificate so that my new birth certificate will show gender (sex) as male, and my name as Zayne. I will then need to change my gender (sex) with the social security office. Once I accomplish these tasks we are planning on being married in June 2008. This will be a legal marriage recognized by the state and federal government because I am male. We don't see this as a bad decision. There are many benefits to being married. I know that we will continue to fight for the right of same-sex couples to marry, even after we are married.

One day we would also like to have kids. This is something we have discussed in length. There are a few ways we can have kids. I told Tami that if we were to use artificial insemination then I didn't want to know the donor. I expressed this because I don't ever want to go through another custody battle. We decided that our options were an unknown donor by means of artificial insemination or adoption. We truly look forward to the day that we are parents to an innocent little baby. We both know that raising another child will be a little confusing since I will always be our daughter's mom, but I will be dad to the new baby. We aren't positive on how we will work it all out but we know we will. I know that when the time comes when we do have a child, we have decided that my transition will not be a secret from this child. We both agree that being honest and loving to our children is the best way to go. I have found that by being honest with my daughter about the world and myself she has learned that not all people are alike and that difference is a good thing. Our world is full of diversity and I believe that we all could learn from one another if we give ourselves that chance.

23

Kayla and Laura

Kayla Karstens

Like all epic love stories, ours is a tale of passion, desire, lust towards others, mistrust, forgiveness, understanding, acceptance, hope, and above all, truth.

My name is Kayla. It is my legal name now but that is not my birth name, nor is female my birth gender. I am a transgendered person. Born male, I've identified with the female gender since the tender age of six, and spent my formative years dressing up in mommy's clothes.

As for my sexual orientation, I see myself as bisexual. Being bisexual is such a powerful position to be in as it allows one the freedom to fall in love with any person and not be influenced by their gender. I dated women, and was even married for six years to a heterosexual woman, who was aware that I was a transgendered person but probably thought all I needed was a good woman. Which she was, but it failed to be a cure and we parted amicably. I've had several serious relationships with gay men and a solitary relationship with a lesbian woman, which was both interesting and exciting since it was not driven by gender attraction but by a mutual S&M fetish. And most recently I am currently in a long-term relationship with another pre-op transgendered person. This is such an interesting relationship with very interesting dynamics.

So what makes this relationship so special or different? Well, plainly put, it's a relationship between two genetically born men who both identify, live, and work in society as women. We regularly have a giggle at how society would view our relationship. Is it gay, since there are still two penises in the bed or are we lesbians since we both identify as women? To date, the consensus is that we see ourselves as "trans-lesbians"; that's the best we can come up with. But what is in a name? And does it really matter since just being transgendered places us way outside most of the boxes that society seems so eager to place us in, or is that place we feel is outside the box just another box?

Geographically, we live in Cape Town, South Africa, a beautiful city nestled on the slopes of Table Mountain. Cape Town is a picturesque postcard city with a sunny climate and expansive white beaches. We are situated right at the tip of Africa, so we have the Atlantic Ocean on our west coast and the Indian Ocean on our east coast and not too far away from where I live, the two oceans collide. This is a beautiful city with a colorful diverse culture, so diverse that we have eleven official languages. But this country also has a dark and oppressive past. South Africa was the home of apartheid. We have only had a democratically elected government since 1994, which is not even a blink in time. I feel it's important that I mention this because most, if not all people, will identify apartheid as the oppression by a minority white government of a black majority, but it actually ran a lot deeper than that.

This was a conservative, Christian-based government that was as oppressive toward gay, lesbian, and transgendered people as it was to people of color. Basically it was against the law not to be heterosexual—not that there were many cases that ever went to court; although sodomy was in the law books as an offence, it was more a case of the police of that time, or even local citizens physically and verbally assaulting trans, gay, and lesbian persons openly in public with no legal consequences if discovered.

However, if a gay, lesbian, or transgendered person ever had the misconception that they could report such an assault to the police in those years, it would normally result in a further abuse, verbal or physical by the authorities, or at best your complaint would just go missing and nothing would ever be done to apprehend those responsible. Being a transgendered person, I was easy to spot in public and so rather than paint a target on my back, I spent most of those years living a double life, changing my clothes and gender roles as and when the opportunity arose. This was a horrid time in my life.

Then in 1994 when South Africa became a democracy under the rule of the African National Congress (ANC) led by Nelson Mandela, our new constitution was introduced that not only gave freedom to people of color but also granted the individual freedom of gender and sexual preference. It became illegal and unconstitutional to discriminate in any way against an individual regarding their race, religious beliefs, sexual preference, and gender. I was finally free to be me. However, even with these freedoms of expression now being legal there are still ongoing hate crimes, and in most of the other African countries trans, gay, and lesbian persons are still legally severely discriminated against, often under threat of imprisonment or worse. Any trans, lesbian, or gay persons reading this account, consider yourself fortunate if you are living in a liberal country like I am; many of our sisters and brothers are not and are paying a high price for their gender and sexual preferences.

Laura, my partner, did not experience much of pre-Apartheid time, since I am forty-two years old and she is twenty-six, an age difference which I find hardly noticeable at times but glaringly apparent at others. I'm getting ahead of myself, so let's backtrack a bit and I'll tell you how we became friends, lovers, and partners.   '

Laura and I met at a transgendered support group meeting one Saturday morning in 2005 and in hindsight we both admitted to being initially drawn to each other. I saw her sitting over the table from me, so young, so innocent; well, maybe not so innocent, but she was gorgeous. One of those trans women who don't seem to have to try to be convincing as a woman. I could not take my eyes off of the black mane of hair falling on her soft shoulders, those huge eyes and that perfect nose; the thoughts that went through my mind that morning, let's just say if I was Catholic I would have spent a whole lot more time in the confessional than normal.

We fast became firm friends, and soon discovered we lived only a few kilometers from each other. Over the next few weeks that turned into months we surpassed being just friends, and I took on the role of being her big sister and we even called each other sisters. So it seemed that the trend of our relationship was set, we would be sisters, close, sharing everything except our bodies, which in hindsight was such a waste. This continued for almost a year. We'd go out to movies, out to dinner, or just spend time together, never crossing that line that would turn our friendship into a sexual relationship. Why, you ask? We both were obviously attracted to each other, and got along well. I suppose it was the idea that with a seventeen-year age difference, a relationship would never work. The big sister role I had assumed seemed to suppress any feelings of sexual attraction; well, not really but that's my story and I'm sticking to it.

We doted on each other. I would do everything in my power to make her journey of transition more painless than mine had been and she was always available to help me through any crisis, to be my sympathetic ear—we both had found a shoulder to lean on. This delicately balanced relationship went on for almost a full year. Then Laura had a crush on another transgendered person, who in turn was not interested in her and she was devastated.

So why are two transgendered people dating each other? The answer is so simple: necessity. Well for us anyway. Despite my bisexual nature, at the time both Laura and I had been interested in men. We both had wonderful adventures dating within the gay community only to find that once the hormones started taking effect, our respective lovers who were gay men rejected us. Why would a gay man who is attracted to other men be the slightest bit interested in a "man" that is trying to be a woman? An effeminate man maybe, but not a man living as a woman. So that was the problem: gay men want real men, straight women want straight men, and lesbian women want other women, and just forget about a straight man showing any interest.

So where does that leave us as pre-op transgendered people? The logical choice is to date another transgendered person who could understand transgendered needs, a fact that I only discovered after being celibate for almost a year, after my last gay boyfriend left me. Allow me to rephrase that. He never just left me; he left running for the hills, repulsed by my pubescent breasts. I cried for weeks. Bye-bye boyfriend, hello loneliness.

There followed a year during which I nearly lost my mind. I love closeness, to touch, to feel, to smell, to taste that special someone. I made various attempts to seek out love and closeness, only to be rejected time and time again.

I believe in some countries there are a multitude of people that are seen as trans lovers. Well I tried and tried but was totally mystified to find that no one I had contact with was vaguely interested in dating a transgendered person, let alone be intimate with and want to start a meaningful relationship with. I blame it on our repressive culture and conservative past in South Africa. My ego screamed, "It surely couldn't be me," since I am gorgeous and fun, artistic, and intelligent, aspects which everyone loves till they find out I'm transgendered.

I had an earlier fling with another transgendered person. This brief affair only lasted two nights, but that flirtation opened my mind to the reality that there are potential lovers among the transgendered community. Up until that point I had never even considered this option, so a door of opportunity swung open, and being bisexual I had no problem with this.

Laura was devastated; she was in love with someone who was not interested. So to cheer her up, big sister—yes that's me if you've forgotten—decided to console her by inviting her to my house for pizza and DVDs. She accepted the invitation, and we drowned our collective sorrows in red wine. I announced that I was too intoxicated to drive her home but that she should phone her father to fetch her. Or spend the night. Believe it or not, this was not a setup; I was truly being big sisterly. I had envisioned us just snuggling up in the same bed and falling asleep quite innocently.

Well I guess you know what followed. We climbed into bed, snuggled up, then Laura (remember what I said earlier about her innocence or lack there of) actually asked me if I mind if we just kiss goodnight. I replied, with the clichéd line: "I'd love to but only if it does not destroy our friendship." What was I thinking? Why did I say that, when in reality I'm such a hedonist and all I wanted to do was be naked next to this gorgeous creature?

Resistance was futile and fleeting. I think before she even responded I kissed her fully on the lips and without hesitation she kissed back. What a wonderful night of passion! The kind of lovemaking that never seems to repeat itself in a relationship, that one night of unbridled passion that ended my year of celibacy. We spent the entire night wrapped in each other, as one being. In the morning I impulsively asked her to move into my house and live with me. I'll give you three guesses what she replied to that? Yes! Yes! Yes! By later that afternoon she had fetched her clothes and moved in. We were so happy; we spent not only the next few hours or the next few days but the next few months inseparable from each other in this fairytale romance.

We were such different people who seemed to bridge those differences without the slightest difficulty. We were no longer alone on our journey into womanhood, but a couple who would share each other's experiences and discoveries. At the start of our intimate relationship, Laura had only been on hormones for about two months, and over the following months I was to watch and feel as these powerful drugs took their effect on her. Over the months as I stroked that gorgeous body of hers I felt her skin soften, and could feel where she was picking up a bit of weight to give her that gorgeous feminine figure she has and watched in amazement as her typically boyish nipples transformed before my eyes. It was a wonderful time for me as an observer, since I'd been taking hormones for two years at this point and the changes had been gradual and not so noticeable to me although I can see the effects clearly when looking at before and after photographs.

There are also huge emotional changes that accompany the physical changes; since I have been on estrogen I have become more at peace with myself and the world. I went through a nasty stage in the years before hormone replacement, where I was for no justifiable reason just angry all the time. I suppose I was taking it out on the world that I was transgendered and in hindsight I cannot believe I used to be that way. The hormones have had such a calming effect on me. You start to realize you are busy with the process of actually doing something about changing your gender, and that in itself is huge.

We have such hugely opposite characters, yet have so much common ground as well. Laura is seventeen years my junior and at twenty-six she is wild and adventurous. She worked for a promotions company which allowed her to work only three days a week most of the year. This gave us lots of time together as I'm a jazz musician, so although I perform five shows a week, I was free all day. We made such good use of that time, seldom apart.

We were both so happy. We became the type of inseparable couple that can drive other people insane with how in love we were, not to mention our public displays of affection, always in each other's arms. I loved every minute of it. I even thought this could be "the one" and was starting to consider changing my will to include this lover of mine. I did not see it coming. On the surface we were the perfect couple but the cracks had started to appear.

So what could drive two people apart who were so obviously in love? Simply the answer was fear of change. My gender reassignment surgery was looming on the horizon. And this affected Laura initially more than it did me, but it was to start affecting me in the following months. It was like opening Pandora's Box—once those fears had been revealed we never could go back to how it was. But what was there to fear? Shouldn't we be happy that my surgery was imminent?

Well first of all, Laura absolutely adores pre-op transgendered women, but is not attracted to post-op transgendered women. And then a factor that I would never have considered: she believes that once I am post-op, she will be envious and even jealous of the fact that I have transitioned while she is still pre-op and this will affect the way she feels toward me. She told me it would make her feel like less of a woman. I was totally shocked by this admission at first but I thought about it for a few days and started to understand where she was coming from. I put it in the context of your best friend graduating and you being left behind for another semester. After surgery we would no longer be equals.

That's from her side but from my side I was also confused. I was not sure how my outlook on relationships would change post-op. Once I have a functional vagina, I will be empowered to have relationships with straight men, or lesbian women, and not be confined to dating transgendered people as I feel I am as a pre-op transgendered person. My prospective dating pool was about to get a whole lot bigger thanks to the surgery.

There was no initial action or reaction once we had discussed these points but it was the hairline crack that would widen over the next few weeks. Then the crack turned into a crevice, when one evening about six months into our relationship, after a social occasion we attended together, she suddenly announced that she was leaving me. This admission caught me so off guard, as in all our time together we'd had only one fight to speak of and I assumed everything was fine. She was saying that she was homesick and missing her family, but in reality they only lived about three kilometers away from where we lived, her parents accepted and approved of our relationship and she was free to visit whenever she liked. So I didn't quite buy that, but it seemed that the main reason was that she was under the impression that she had a chance of dating the person that she had initially been infatuated with. Lust . . . as a hedonist, I can understand lust. So we broke up. I was devastated, and absolutely amazed that I had not seen it coming. Being older and wiser, or possibly just more foolish, I just let it go; no fighting, no begging, just surrender. The logic being that you cannot force someone to love you. We never spoke for a week, a week in which I reflected on what had happened and had come to realize that the underlying problems of me being so close to being post-op was more to blame than anything else; she knew she would be losing me in a few months, so why not grab an opportunity for sex and a possible relationship with a young, beautiful transgendered person whom she is obviously infatuated with and someone who was also a few years from transitioning.

Almost a week to the day we visited each other; needless to say, Laura's infatuation with that other person never came to fruition, not even resulting in a one-night stand, so the hedonist in me came to the fore once more. I agreed that I was not sure whether I wanted another live-in relationship with her, but we could be friends who were intimate with each other. We called it "inappropriate friends," but I was later to learn the accepted term for this is "friends with benefits." I'd like to think that this move was motivated not by desperation or loneliness but out of love, a love I obviously felt for her. However, all the drama of the current potential affair and the impending doom of the upcoming surgery dates certainly put a unique spin on the problem and how we were to solve it?

I was initially adamant that I would not get into a relationship with her again as I was still quite emotionally wounded by the break-up. And surely it must be a case of once bitten twice shy. But I am not the strong-willed woman I thought I was. Us being "friends with benefits" only lasted a few weeks but as I held her and smelt her and touched her, all resistance to being in a relationship with her again was lost. I once more surrendered and even though I must admit there was a small amount of mistrust of her on my mind, we were once more a couple.

Surgery was creeping ever nearer, and to finance the surgery I had to sell the only valuable asset I possessed: my house. I was not happy but what could I do? I'm not getting any younger, and at forty-two and being a musician, I simply could not afford to transition any other way. The sale of the house placed much strain on the relationship. I became like a bear with a sore head at times; the stress mounted as I needed to sell the house quickly as I had already been communicating for months with Dr. Suporn in Thailand to perform both my gender and facial feminizing surgery. The Suporn clinic is so popular it is booked up at least six months in advance, so the sale was urgent to reserve a surgery date, which eventually became March 21, 2007 for my gender surgery and April 4, 2007 for my facial feminization surgery. At last my surgery dates were set. But in this chaotic and stressful time leading up to the sale and the confirmation of my surgery, there was to be more drama, and I must take partial blame because of my overstressed state during this time.

Before I continue, I have to wonder, how do people who are less fortunate than me afford to transition? Although South Africa has a sufficiently transgendered friendly constitution and legal system, it has all but stopped any government-funded programs for gender reassignment. The idea of a public health system for transgendered or in fact any financially challenged persons is totally inefficient or even nonexistent as in the case of gender reassignment surgery. We have replaced racial apartheid in this country with financial apartheid. I am the living proof of that since I had to sell a house to achieve my transition. I am aware it is a bad financial decision but I have no other options available to me, but then I get even more depressed when I realize that many transgendered people like me don't even have a home to sell. I'll step down from my soap box and continue our story now. However, all these social and political issues are very much a part of our story and cannot be ignored as it has influenced us both so radically in the decisions we make as transgendered persons and as partners.

As they say in all the classics, "the plot thickens" once more. Like that moth drawn to the flame, I was to be burnt yet again. Oh yes, believe it or not by the same infatuation; once more Laura believed she could achieve her conquest with that very same person with whom she has been infatuated since before our relationship had even started. And once more it was to be fruitless. This time I was more hurt than the first, but after a lot of begging on her part to resume our relationship, I decided that we could continue; however, it would never be that unconditional love that was there all those months ago.

So twice bitten, yet amazingly the power of human touch triumphed once more and we resumed a rather unique relationship that for all intents and purposes had become an open relationship with the understanding that with only a few months to my surgery in March 2007 and the imminent end of us being lovers, we should not live together but just spend one or two nights a week together and be free to end the relationship at any time if someone else were to appear a more attractive offer to either of us, the agreement being we would end it with each other before pursuing other conquests. Mostly because we are both very HIV-conscious and when we tested together both of us tested negative and we want to retain that status. The only rule in our relationship was to be honest with each other and if we transgress to admit it immediately to each other.

Well that was a few months ago and so far we're still being intimate and spending a day or two a week together. I have moved into a new home, a house I share with an artist and human rights activist, Gabrielle Le Roux. This relationship between Gabrielle and I has inspired an art project and a possible documentary which will record me through my transition before, during, and after surgery, with various art works in various mediums, oil paintings, charcoal drawings, and pastels.

We have already spent many glorious summer afternoons up in Gabrielle's studio with the warm sunlight streaming. It is a wonderful space in which Laura and I, always totally naked, snuggle up to each other on the bed and find some pose that Gabrielle would like to draw; invariably we are embraced in each other's arms and all the drawings show the closeness that is between us. It is such an intimate time and despite the fact that we are not alone and are being drawn, we are both totally comfortable with each other and Gabrielle. It feels as natural to us as any two lovers snuggled up in bed together on a Sunday morning. We spend the time caressing each other, kissing, and chatting softly.

I think Laura and I are getting more out of these art sessions than just the art; it's a documentation of our relationship that will be immortalized in Gabrielle's art. It's quite interesting to think that many years, even decades, or maybe even centuries from now, someone will look at these works of art and possibly wonder about the two transgendered people who are featured in so many of Gabrielle le Roux's works over this time period. Our relationship immortalized.

So why is this relevant? Because at the time of this writing we have about six or seven works of original art by Gabrielle Le Roux of Laura and I. We have a drawing session at least once a week. So the art project is not only documenting my transition but also my relationship with Laura, which despite the ups and downs is still going strong. With only just over two months until my surgery we are still together, and I would venture a guess that we will still be together until I am post-op. Probably not after that, but what an achievement given the circumstances. This is surely a testament to how love can survive bizarre situations.

And talking about love and bizarre situations, I've saved the description of our sex life until the end. Sexually we are two raving animals, but only in our heads. Well the truth is that due to the effect of the testosterone blocker we both take as part of our hormone regime, it renders us pretty much useless to enjoy sex in the usual manner. The amazing fact is that our sex drive is still perfectly intact and if we could physically act on our thoughts we'd be an awesome sexual couple. Instead we are huge on touching, holding, caressing, and kissing.

We both share the same endocrinologist so we both seem to experience the same physical constraints, which seem to vary among transgendered persons. Since being on the hormones and the testosterone blocker we both are sexually stimulated but neither is able to achieve, let alone sustain, an erection for long enough to enjoy any form of penetrative sex. This lack of sexual performance has been replaced by a closeness that is incredible; we can lie in each other's arms for hours, we sleep embraced, always touching caressing, nibbling, stroking. We both miss not having orgasms but are finding ways to touch and feel wonderful without it. Nevertheless, having an orgasm is the one pleasure I cannot wait to reclaim once I have my new vagina. We still both enjoy the intense connection that we built on love, possibly out of desperation, but a relationship that amazingly held together even through several dramas and temptations. We sense the future, anticipate it, even accept the inevitable, but still find a warm safe place in each other's arms.

I'm so glad to have met Laura when I did; she has been instrumental in allowing me to approach my surgery with the feeling of being loved. I have spoken and interacted with many transgendered persons who have faced this last leg of the journey alone, divorced from spouses, or separated from same-sex partners; lonely, scared, desperately in need of the touch of a lover, someone to whisper in your ear that regardless of what obstacles we face, everything will be just perfect. At the time of this writing I'm in that very place, scared of my unknown future, even more scared of the pain of surgery, and the thought of losing a lover because of the surgery. I'm so fortunate that when I awaken in the middle of the night and the darkness seems to be closing in on me, I have Laura to hold me close and whisper in my ear that everything will be just perfect.

This is dedicated to Laura.

24

Madam Carmen

Carmen Rupe

My name is Carmen Rupe and I'm from the beautiful country of New Zealand. I am Maori, with some English and French ancestors thrown in, from the Ngati Maniopoto tribe in the king country town of Taumarunui. My father's tribe was Maniopoto and my mother's Ngati Haua. I was actually born Trevor David Rupe but somewhere along the way to my seventy-plus years young, I became Carmen, New Zealand's first famous out-and-out transsexual striptease artist.

I remember my lovely mother Elsie as being a very beautiful, tall, and extremely house-proud woman but she died at forty-five when I was in my early teens. I only know my father John from his pictures as I really have very little memory of him and it was my grandparents who raised us after my mother died. I have some brief memories of my father's farm, then my mother's house but the center of my young life was on my grandfather's farm at the end of a dirt road with no electricity. My family has always been very protective and even if someone would say an unkind thing about me, my family would always support me and put them in their place.

I still feel close to my mother's spirit and often talk to her, make some cakes for her, and encourage her to eat them. I can feel close to other spirits of my family, like grandparents, aunties, uncles, my siblings who have passed on, and cousins who I feel are not far away in the great beyond. Maori culture can be quite close. We have extended families and we believe all our kinfolk are not far away. We make welcome even people who we have not met if they are from our family.

My father was a hard-working man and we lived on his farm with the usual extended Maori family of aunts, uncles, and cousins. If you are Maori there are so many cousins, even if you are not related by blood to them. Unfortunately, my father was also a very jealous and possessive man. When I was five, my mother fell for another man and father shot himself.

My family has always been so loving to me. I remember us being very close, so I guess I have been lucky that way. We were a family of three sisters and seven brothers and to begin with, I was one of the boys and then later one of the girls. When I was born, my mother wanted a girl so she dressed me up very feminine and I got to do many of the things that girls did. We lived with my mother and grandparents and it did not matter what you were; there was so much love in our family that I always felt valued. I realized when I was young that I was different from all the other boys, although it was not until I was a teenager that I found out how different I really was. My family believed in "live and let live" so my family ties have stayed strong all throughout the years, even to this day.

As a child I was my mother's helper; I learned to calculate every penny of the shopping money since it was rations in the 1940s after the Second World War and everything had to add up. This helped me tremendously in later years when I was a successful business woman running my own nightclubs and a coffee bar in Wellington. I suppose I was New Zealand's first out public transsexual and wherever you went, everyone seemed to know my name.

I started my professional career in drag as a female impersonator in Sydney's Kings Cross, Australia in 1958 doing belly dancing and dancing with snakes. Of course it was all illegal and run by the Mafia but in those days you were just a queen that got on with things. The Cross was a fascinating place full of sex workers, drag queens, male whores, curb crawlers, transvestites, strippers, and dancers. It was an exciting place to be the first Maori drag queen from New Zealand.

I worked in clubs such as the Jewel Box as a female impersonator and then, when the famous Australian drag queen Carlotta opened Les Girls, I went to work there. I had an act as a Hawaiian hula dancer and, since I was Maori, the tourists could not tell the difference. Then as I got better known I graduated to a glamorous striptease act. That place sure was an education, as the bars and cafés were open twenty-four hours a day if they were paying the right heavies. The police were tough on drag queens and prostitutes back in the 1960s. I was also one of the regular performers at Sydney's first gay bar called the Purple Onion. As a drag queen if you got caught with ladies' underwear on, you ran the risk of being arrested and sent to prison. The drag queens worked William Street which was a meeting point for them and their clients. Most of them had their tits done or the full change. It was a time of glamour queens. Kings Cross was buzzing and you would often get customers in Rolls Royces pulling up looking for some action.

Working for four years in Cornwall Hospital in Auckland and a year in Sydney's Concord Hospital, as a male nurse, I had learned to direct and manage people. I had also spent a year at the age of eighteen conscripted into the New Zealand army so I did not frighten that easy and things were so corrupt that the police took bribes to leave us alone.

I was never a great smoker, drug-taker, or fall-down drunk, but I loved to put on a show and have a party so people could have a good time. As a nightclub owner or a madam I always treated my staff very well and I think many of them remember me as a friend. That's just my way. I've always thought of myself as a public person and when it was all still illegal I was an advocate for transsexuals, sex workers, and legal abortion. Being a bisexual person, I was even more different in those days for a transsexual. I suppose because I had so much unconditional love when I was young, it gave me the confidence and courage to just be who I am.

Once I was sent to prison for nine months when I was twenty-two for running what I used to call a "Kind House of Entertainment," but I still came out loving the world. They were so nice to me in prison and let me out after six months because I had spent most of the time making the governor lots of cups of tea all day long.

When I was seventeen I went on holiday to Auckland and happened to meet a man who was much older then me. I was very innocent. We had dinner and drinks and I really thought we were just having a platonic relationship. It seems I had more drinks than dinner. Back at his apartment he photographed me naked, and after getting me even more drunk, ensured I was innocent no more. It was the ruin of me because after that I was man crazy and that is how I've been ever since.

There was a girl when I was nineteen, though. She was really pretty like the English actress Diana Dors and such a lovely person. I was quite taken with her big time but when I started to cross-dress and do drag she could not really cope with it and it put her off me. I don't know what happened to her but I often think about her and have her picture on my wall.

Men were my real passion. Before I started to live full time as a female, I would hang around in the gay bars, which were often secret rooms at the back of hotels in those days. I would also go down to the docks with friends in New Zealand and we would pick up the sailors.

When I became a cabaret star and lived full time as female, men went nuts for me. They seemed to be absolutely fascinated. I suppose there were not that many of us around in those days so we probably had a larger fascination factor and mystique. I was dark and sultry and really enjoyed playing the sexy siren. I think I truly was Bizet's Carmen. I was not like many of the other trans girls as I never wanted to meet just one man and settle down. I like variety and lots of it. The more men the better and it's not something I've ever been ashamed of because I'm just me and I wanted to share it around.

I was always attracted to two kinds of men and both of them white. I'm not racist; it's just my thing. I like rugged, handsome types like the film star Marlon Brando—cute with muscles. You know, looks, but not too much thinking. My second penchant was for smart businessmen in suits who had lots of money and power who wanted to have a good time. As long as they could provide the money, I could always provide the good time.

My International Coffee Lounge in Wellington had five bedrooms upstairs and they were certainly not for drinking coffee. I was renowned as Madam Carmen and I earned it but all the boys, girls, and trannies who worked for me were very happy and we were a family. The customers had a code whereby they would place their cup in three different positions to indicate whether they wanted a boy, girl, or something in between. Yes, I was always getting fined and appearing in the newspapers, but let's be honest, what is paid to the courts eventually comes back around to sex workers' purses. "Business" as they say, "is business," no matter which side of the bench you sit on.

I have fallen in love often and for brief periods but when a guy wanted to get too serious, I wanted to get someone else. There were two men, however, who I was quite in love with. One was a New Zealand All Blacks rugby player and the other a very famous cricketer. I have always sworn I would never reveal their names; after all, like the rest, they were married and had families. By now they would be grandfathers and I would not want to embarrass their families with me being so well known.

In the 1950s I took hormone pills which really feminized me and in the early 1970s I had breast augmentations. So I'm a brass with a rack. And what a rack, as I never do anything by halves. I never had genital surgery, though, and believe me, the men did not actually mind. For some of them it was the cherry on the cake and I was the most colorful cake in the shop.

I thought about having a vagina and many of my friends went off to Egypt to a surgeon who was operating there. I even arranged a visit but then President Nasser was assassinated, everything in Egypt changed, and they rang me and told me not to come. After that I just did not bother with the idea. Not having a vagina never really held me back. The hormones shrank everything down there and there's a lot you can do for your money without assuming the missionary position.

I've been a nurse, soldier, male prostitute, night club bouncer, drag queen, striptease artist, cabaret act, madam, night club owner, businesswoman, and street hustler, and enjoyed the lot. I never looked down on anyone and I hope in their kindness, people have the good grace not to look down on me either. I truly have loved rather than hated, even if I often charged for it, but you can bet the services I have provided have saved a good few marriages. Let's be honest, men rarely get everything they want at home and what they want is generally a good time.

For a great part of my life I was a girl who had love for sale and with many of those customers it might have been the only love they were actually receiving. Some readers may want me to divide love from sex or sex from love but I don't think that is always possible, even if is bought or hired love. Let's just say I did a lot of social work for a lot of men over a lot of years.

It's not that I was more beautiful than those men's wives. It's just that I was more available, looked like a fantasy figure, was ready for instant gratification, never told tales, was always happy to see them, did things their wives wouldn't, was less expensive in the long run, available for short-term engagements and was always good value for the money. I generally loved them by the hour with the meter running. It's not callous, crass, or unkind. It is, in fact, the opposite because everyone wants to be loved and often paying for it by the hour is far less expensive than having to pay for it for the rest of your life.

So did my father shooting himself when I was five or my mother dying when I was a young teenager damage my confidence in the idea of long-term relationships? No, I really don't think it did. My grandfather was a tribal healer and my grandmother also had a wonderful healing aura. My brothers and sisters always loved me and I always felt wanted. You see, because I had so much love at home, I was not a butterfly flying from flower to flower out of fear, but out of choice.

There is little doubt I've been a people's person and taken part in the community using my fame and notoriety to open things and help people by raising money for charity when I can. Because I've kept myself glamorous and always dressed very well, I suppose I've been a very popular celebrity. People expect that as a show person you look glamorous when they meet you, so I try not to disappoint.

Since I was so well known I had to be very discreet about some of my lovers' names. In the 1970s I ran for the Mayor of Wellington and came in second. If I had been a blabbermouth there would have been a lot of wives not voting for me. My mayoral campaign was "Vote For Carmen: Get in behind."

Even when I wrote my autobiography, *Carmen: My Life from Schoolboy to Successful Business Woman* back in the 1980s I was discreet about the men I named. I tried not to cause any divorces because if I had told about all the men I've known, the courts would have been busy to bursting. Sure, there were lots of MPs and local socialites and dignitaries who came to my clubs in New Zealand. I even went to parliament myself for a visit once in a chauffeur-driven limousine. I had been called before the bar of the New Zealand House of Parliament to explain why I had publicly said there were homosexual MPs and sure enough, the truth eventually changed things. New Zealand today is one of the world's most progressive countries on human rights. They did not invite me to stay to lunch, though; maybe they were afraid I would serve up a little too much kiss-and-tell for desert.

I had a big seventieth birthday party in Sydney recently and one in New Zealand with lots of my friends and family. It was lovely to see everyone and because I was so famous I'm still treated like a celebrity, being honored at the 2002 opening of the Sydney Gay Games.

Today I am semi-retired and live alone in a small apartment in Sydney's Surry Hills. It is a queer and fashionable sort of district that used to be associated with gangsters and brothels. In fact, there are still brothels here right across the road from my door. I run a little social center in the block of units where I live. Because I was one of the lights that lit up Kings Cross just around the corner, I guess you could say I'm never very far from home.

Is there anything that I regret? Well, I never had children. I look at mothers in the street with their children and wish I had been born female so I could have had lots of kids. I think I would have been a good mother, but with my wandering eye I'm so not sure I could have been a good wife. Well, not faithful anyway. I would have had thirteen children. That's six boys, six girls, and of course one in between.

Every Sunday I go to church and ask God and Jesus to forgive me for any wicked things I have done. Maybe some day I'll still find myself a nice sugar daddy to keep me in the kind of luxury I am really accustomed to, or would that be still more sin? Oh well . . . I never could say no to a little more sin, or maybe a lot if the opportunity arises.

25

Still Queer After All These Years: Reflections on Being in a Trans Couple

Joelle Ruby Ryan

Many years ago, I remember seeing a tabloid at the grocery store. As my mother started to place food on the check-out counter, I took down the rag and started to look at the story, which intrigued my fourteen-year-old eyes. The headline blared "British couple swap sexes!" and the article talked about the couple who started off as a conventional man and woman and ended up in "reverse" gender roles. The story included pictures of the transsexual coupling, and though sensationalistic in tone, I remember feeling excited to see the story. There was a whole world of people like me out there, and they were even forming families!

In the early 1990s, I remember seeing the cover of a transvestite-transsexual (TV-TS) magazine which featured a male-to-female and female-to-male transsexual couple on the cover. At a trans forum I was at, the presenter held up the magazine and tried to explain the cover to an increasingly confused audience. Finally, in exasperation, she pointed to the FTM and said "girl" (referring to the person's pre-transition sex) and then pointed to the MTF and said "boy" and then said the word "couple." The crowd started shaking their heads and emitting "wows" and "no ways" galore. Once again, my mind was opened to a new possibility.

Shortly thereafter, I remember renting the film *It's Pat: The Movie.* I had always found the Pat comedy bits on *Saturday Night Live* to be offensive and sophomoric. But there is something about the movie that just tugs at my heart strings. I think it is the relationship between

Trans People In Love

Pat (Julia Sweeney) and Chris (Dave Foley) that manages to be sweet and tender, despite its one-joke overload. Even if Pat is a nerdy, socially-inept goofball, the fact that s/he is shown in a caring and loving relationship with Chris is significant, for through this coupling s/he is rendered lovable and therefore human. The best part of the film is that Pat's "true" gender is never revealed, thus reaffirming Pat's right to live a fluid, genderqueer existence.

In the late 1990s, well after I had come out as a male-to-female trans woman, I remember being on a panel and being asked about relationships. The professor who was facilitating the panel for her class somewhat prophetically asked me if I would ever date an FTM. At the time I kind of shrugged my shoulders, because to be honest I had not given much thought to the idea. Most of my life I had been asexual, and did not have a clearly defined attraction to "men" or "women." I think I had given up on the notion of a relationship, because as a 6'6" trans woman who was not easily identifiable in the terms of the gender binary: male/female, masculine/feminine, gay/straight, I felt like an eternal misfit.

But this all changed in the Fall of 2003. I had just moved to Bowling Green, Ohio to start a doctoral program in American Studies at Bowling Green State University (BGSU). Bowling Green is a very rural community in Northwest, Ohio, about a half-hour drive from Toledo. The campus of BGSU has around 20,000 students, but it is not particularly diverse. This is especially true in regards to gender identity and gender expression. As I began my graduate student orientation and looked around at all the cookie-cutter men and women, a veritable plethora of "Chips" and "Buffys," I worried that my depression would worsen due to lack of opportunities to socialize with other trans and genderqueer folks in the area. I knew there were at least a few trannies in the area because they had sent e-mails to me when I was considering coming to the school.

One of those folks who had written me was Brandon, a twenty-five-year-old FTM who had received his BA from BGSU and currently worked on campus for Instructional Media Services, helping faculty with their classrooms' technology needs. Some folks strongly believe in love at first sight. I am not one of them. My first impression of Brandon was that he seemed like a very mellow and sweet person. I was also thrilled to meet another trans person in the area. But for me there were no lightning strikes or thunder bolts during that first interaction. I merely hoped to make a friend and find some sense of trans community in the area.

Our relationship proceeded very slowly. For our first, unofficial "date" we attended the Bowling Green Black Swamp Arts Festival. We looked at art and jewelry, drank homemade lemonade, ate French fries, and enjoyed the warm weather and each other's company. It would not be until nearly three months later that our relationship began to have a physical component. I thank the heavens that Brandon made the first "move," because otherwise our relationship may have never gotten off the ground! Luckily, our mutual friend Amy served as an excellent matchmaker. What we were too scaredy-cat to say to each other, we would say to Amy, who would transmit the message.

I approached so much of the relationship with fear and trepidation. As a 6'6" nonpassing trans woman who has lived in rural areas her whole life, my life has been one battle after another. From familial rejection, to constant economic problems, to the terror of street-level abuse and harassment, I have not had an easy time of it. I marvel at the difference between me now and me as a freshman undergrad. Back then, I approached the world with so much more openness, wide-eyed innocence, and positive anticipation. Since then, I have become more cynical, more jaded and bitter, and more world-weary. Some people have pretty smooth transitions; mine has felt difficult at every turn. The biggest thing I have lost is the ability to trust people, to see them as natural allies. I think when you get fucked over so much, it is easy to become guarded and aloof.

From my perspective, the hardest thing that Brandon has had to do is to melt through the layers of ice. I can put up walls like nobody's business. It is a protective mechanism to keep the innermost parts of me safe and inviolate. Like the stone butch figure, my body becomes stone to keep the cruelty of the world at bay. But through dogged determination, Brandon has melted his way through to the inner core, and I honestly feel better than ever before in my life. While I worried endlessly about being exposed and vulnerable, I actually feel stronger and more powerful. I don't let many people in, and through inviting Brandon into my inner emotional world, I feel like a giant burden has been lifted from my spirit.

Part of that burden is letting go of easy notions of identity and sexuality. Whenever I would do a panel about being trans, people would ask me if I was attracted to "men" or "women." I would always hum and haw, and usually tell them that I was some variation of bisexual or pansexual. Now I understand that my response was not the problem; the problem lies in the question itself. I think that the question, for me at least, is unintelligible. Sex, gender, and sexuality are far too complex to be placed in a binary system. This is true for everyone, but it is especially true for trans people.

The system of sexual orientation we employ in the U.S. is based on compliance with gender norms and on Western, dichotomous thinking. It is rooted in the assumption that biological sex matches one's gender identity, gender identity matches one's gender expression, and that one is solely attracted to men OR women. The trans, intersex, and genderqueer movements for liberation have challenged traditional notions of sex, gender, and sexuality and have forwarded a radical agenda based on diversity and empowerment. The body, gender, and sexual longing cannot be contained by hegemonic ideology, nor can they be universally described by either/or, black-or-white identity labels.

The gender police wish to put everyone in a culturally-legible box. One of the things I love about my relationship is that we will not allow people to do that to us. While Brandon comes out of the lesbian community, I come out largely of the gay male community. As we join together as a couple, does that now make us straight? Hell no! We were queer then and we are queer now. Our sexuality is not based on our biological sex or even on our gender identities/expressions. It is based on our own self-definitions and ways of identifying in relation to the larger social world.

After dating for about a year, I remember us walking down the street in Bowling Green holding hands. A car went by and somebody craned their head out to yell: "Is that your boyfriend or your girlfriend?" While at the time I was angered at the rude bigotry, now I see humor in the incident. I did not know if they were addressing their comment to me or to Brandon! Many years ago, a trans woman friend and I went out to eat after a late night of clubbing at a Goth bar. Some drunken frat guys noticed us right away and begin to yell insults at our table. The coup de grace was when one of them stepped up to our table and asked which one of us played the "man" and which one played the "woman." Genderism, heterosexism, and misogyny are so deep-seated in our culture that strangers feel the need to place people in their sexual straight jackets. Both incidents reveal how threatened people are by those individuals and couples who stray from the boundaries of gender and sexual normativity.

This societal intolerance and uneasiness was also confirmed by the rude questions some people asked me when they found out about Brandon and I being together. "Well, how does *that* work?" "How do you guys have sex?" The more puzzled people became, the more I began to think about the stultifying and unyielding nature of the sex/gender system. If we are truly going to support gender and sexual liberation, then that means coming to terms with configurations that makes us uncomfortable, anxious, or even baffled. It means allowing people the space to identify, dis-identify or *not* identify in accordance with their genuine sense of self rather than our preconceived notions. It means the right to ambiguity, changeability, indecisiveness, fluidity, and multiplicity.

When people at the mall in our conservative community look at Brandon and I, they don't usually think: "Aw shucks, what a cute straight couple!" They more likely think: "What is this, what is that, and what on earth are they doing kissing each other on the lips?" Certainly this can be trying and frustrating at times, but I honestly value being a part of the cutting-edge sex/gender frontier. Through our queerness and unique permutations of sex and gender, we are forging our own mini-revolution, moving the culture forward in the continuous deconstruction of sexuality and the proliferation of freedom and liberation. And, for the record, *it* works just fine!

The love that Brandon has brought into my life is valuable beyond measure. I have become a better person in so many ways through our relationship. I am not one to privilege monogamous pair-bonding in the romantic sense of it. Nor do I believe that a sexual relationship is inherently more powerful or transformative than a platonic one. But I do believe that certain people, in whatever relationship to us, can change our lives for the better and make us healthier human beings. Brandon has helped a part of me shine that was always hidden in the shadows before, and for this I am eternally grateful.

In addition, I love the way we "queer" notions of gender and sexuality in our community and in our culture. In a world always asking for simplistic answers, just through daring to be together we throw assumptions to the wind and demand that people acknowledge us as full human beings with integrity rather than as immoral freaks or walking identity labels.

As the tagline for *Pat: The Movie* states, love really is a many gendered thing, and I feel honored to be walking that movement forward with my transgender brother, fellow warrior, and beloved. Walking alone, I face so much adversity from the world for being a 6'6", 350-lb trannie of indeterminate gender. But when I am with Brandon, I can lean on his 5'3" frame and feel stronger, for I know that the purity of our love and connection surpasses any ignorant comment or dirty look that comes our way.

As transgender warriors multiplied by two, our loving embrace provides an impenetrable shield to hatred, bigotry, and intolerance. To the person who shouted "Is that your boyfriend or your girlfriend?" I finally have generated a response: "Yes. No. Maybe. It doesn't matter. We are too in love and having way too much fun together to notice." I dream of a world where it really doesn't make a damn bit of difference, where unconditional love has the final word. I believe we *can* make it happen, one mini-revolution at a time.

26

Notes for Trans People

Tracie O'Keefe

Well here we are. I am guessing you have read through the stories by the time you come to this part of the book. I hope you enjoyed them as much as Katrina and I did. So what did you get from them?

I bet every single one of you got something different from them. I am certain though that you all admired the people who shared their stories about being trans and in love. Some of the journeys were easier than others, but we can all celebrate our own successes and we all have to face our own demons. When you are socially pegged as society's misfits, liberation only arrives out of invention.

I have always been fascinated by how the trans and intersex community find new ways of eking out a living, finding a social niche or rallying for equal rights. I have also taken my hat off many times in respect to the loved ones of those people who have stood shoulder to shoulder with them against prejudice and demonstrated their own ability to love.

For so long we have been portrayed as oddities that have a dreadful illness often referred to loosely, and inaccurately, as gender dysphoria. People in white coats spend hours pontificating over exactly which mental disorder we have and how inept they think we may be through life. At the very best we are lumped into the sad and dysfunctional label and at the very worst we are legally deprived of the human rights to make our own choices about our lives. I make no excuses for being a revolutionary. How about you?

I have been in love so many times in my life with deep emotion, passion, trust, lust, and so on. My lovers, boyfriends, and lesbian partners have enriched my life beyond my wildest expectations. For forty years I have abandoned the mediocre expectations of my parents, clinicians, and society in general. I refused to wait for love, opened my heart wide and swallowed every opportunity for love and passion that came my way.

You see, when I first started appearing as female in public, back in 1966, at eleven years old, I discovered that my very existence was offensive to society; so I made up my mind that I had nothing to gain by being coy. When you are eleven on the front of the newspaper, pegged as a freak and everyone at school knows it, it is unlikely you are ever going to reach normality—whatever that is. Sure, I was stealth for a large part of my life without people knowing about my background as a woman of transsexed origin but I reckoned my gynecology was my own damn business. Nowadays the world and their wife know that I am a woman of transsexed background and I have to tell you that is a very comfortable place for me to be. As the fabulous American trans punk rock pioneer Jayne County sang: "If you don't want to fuck me baby, baby fuck off."

Even as a therapist I know I don't have a hope in hell of fitting in the norm. Many clinicians who tout themselves as respectable do not want to work with me or share patients with me because I am the therapist who just happens to be publicly trans. Every year my office gets lunatic letters from people who believe that I shouldn't be practicing and every year they give me more reasons to practice. The intelligent and trusted clinicians and academics that I do work with have already weeded themselves out as thinkers and doers by the very fact they are happy to work with me, and the trans thing is just not an issue.

ARE YOU WITH US OR AGAINST US?

I cannot say mine was an easy journey because it was not. My family deserted me as a teenage trans girl and I was left homeless without any love or support from them. The clinician I was under was a monster and drove me to attempt suicide more times than I care to remember. It was my friends and my lovers that kept me housed and fed until I learned to find my own feet as an adult. Those great loves of my youth bolstered my sense of self and gave me hope that perhaps I just might be more than I was aware of at the time.

Every time I fell in love it was a verification that perhaps I was not the reject society made me out to be. Today I do not need to be in love for self-validation but I have been in love and lived with the same woman for fifteen years. It has been my longest relationship and I think that was because we were friends for two years prior to being lovers. Like me, she is a provocateur and social dissident. I suspect it is the revolutionary in me that she is in love with just as much as the woman.

This has been a different kind of love for me because she is the opposite of the kind of person I thought I would end up with. We are so different in so many ways yet I always feel she is my greatest ally. To be together we have to think outside the box and create a life neither of us thought we would have lived, and it works. I have learned not to give up what I am to get what I want and I know if I did, she would not be interested.

SO WHAT ABOUT MY GENDER DYSPHORIA?

Well, to be honest I never had gender dysphoria. I was always comfortable being female but my genitals as I grew up were in contradiction to what I turned out to be (sex dysphoric). When that was fixed by surgery, I learned to get on with life. Of course I made some mistakes because my development as a person had been arrested due to the delayed arrival of a vagina. I had to grow up as an adult in the way I should have been able to do as a teenager.

Although everyone knows I am transsexed simply by looking on the Internet, it is just not an issue for me anymore. It is more of a historical fact like having gone to such and such a school or so and so college. So many people that come into my office pre- and post-transition have got their trans status way out of proportion. It has become larger than life and sometimes their whole life. When they learn to shrink that part of their life back into a manageable portion it clears the way to carry on with the journey of living and relate to lovers as a person and not simply a "trannie." Of course I jump up and down on protest marches, write papers, give talks and write letters for trans equal rights but then I go home for tea, water the garden, and if I'm lucky, make love with Katrina. In the middle of folding the sheets, cleaning the car, and putting a color on my next-door neighbor's hair, being trans is the very last thing on my mind.

WHAT IF I'M TOO TALL, SMALL, OR MAYBE DON'T PASS?

My mother is to blame . . . I have told her time and time again if she had not had big thighs then I would not have had legs like a Steinway piano. And we laugh because after fifty-two years of being trans and having a mother who has a trans daughter, we have learned to laugh. She complains about the sleepless nights I gave her and I complain about the legs she gave me.

Too fat . . . too thin . . . too short . . . too old . . . too masculine . . . too feminine, some people are just looking for reasons to keep others at arm's length. Life is so short and then it's gone in an instant. I can't promise you that everything in the garden will be rosy because let's face it there are generally thorns where there are roses. But if you don't take a leap of faith, no one will ever want to fall in love with you.

For many of us, being in love in life is not just the icing on the cake, it is the very ingredient that holds the whole thing together. If I die before Katrina I want her to fall in love again. If we don't stay together in the future I would still wish her love, passion, and fire in her soul wherever she may find them.

IS THE MYTH OF THE LONELY TRANS OR INTERSEX PERSON DISSOLVING?

The answer is yes. Many of us have now lived the large majority of our lives as trans. Although that has often caused us legal and social problems, with laws in many places still not allowing us to marry, adopt children, or have equal social space; we have found ways around the prejudice, oppression, and stigma to emerge as rounded human beings. Not only have we changed many laws to give us more equal rights we have shown that being trans does not necessarily mean being a victim. In fact, for many of us it has now become the journey of choice and not just of desperation.

If I had my time over again, would I have chosen to have been born and registered female at birth? The answer is no. I have had an amazing journey with all the roses and the thorns having shaped me. Would I if I could give up being me? Absolutely not, because that would mean giving up all the friends, lovers, and partners I have had and there have been a lot. And when I'm old, gray, and decrepit with senility robbing me of my memories of love, lust, and lamentation, will I want to carry on? No.

So what hope is there for you, my fellow trans traveler in love? Hope, as I always say, is for the nuns ... If you want a loving relationship you need to be responsible for your end of the bargain. Open your heart and be available to welcome in someone who may be special to you. If you have a closed heart, then no one will knock at your door. Take a chance, which could end in success but also carries with it the danger of not working out. Be realistic and be a giver, not just waiting around for someone to come along and make you happy.

It is OK to make the first move and flirt. Remember, you are not just a category in a diagnostic and statistical manual—you are a person. Beauty is borne out of who you are, not just how many facelifts you've had or the number of whiskers on your chin. If it does not work out, pick yourself up and try again with someone else. Treat each journey into love as a learning experience and treasure the journey as much as the end result. And if you have a fabulous time in love, don't be shy, and show the world how love can be done well, with sincerity and bravado.

ODE TO KATRINA

Love is the light that shows the way
Love is the light that makes the day
Love is the passion that raises the moon
Love is the inspiration to sing and croon

Love is my heart that belongs to you
Love is my reason to be true
Love is my prize for being so brave
Love is my last thought in the grave

Love is all we can leave behind
Love is to search and then to find
Love is because I took a chance
Love is your everlasting glance

Love is what you gave to me
Love is our reason to live and be

Love is like your endless kiss
Love like yours is always bliss

May you fall in love just because you can . . .

Lots of love
Tracie and Katrina

27

Notes for Therapists

Tracie O'Keefe

I completed the pilot study for this project back in 2002 when I qualitatively interviewed six couples with at least one person who was trans or intersexed. My intention was to find out how they operated successful relationships under such circumstances; and what were the stumbling blocks that endangered those relationships. The couples were very different but the common theme I concluded was that the success or failure of the relationships appeared largely due to the flexibility of the other partner's adaptability to the person's trans identity.

Although the six couples were only a small sample group, the interviews were mostly in person and structured to help participants reveal their relationship coping strategies. A lot of my observations were based on how the couple interacted in nonverbal ways as well as how they answered questions and how open were the explanations they offered about their relationships. Both of the partners were interviewed together.

In deciding on where to take my investigations, I decided to go back to my original roots as a Rogerian listener. One of the problems with being a researcher in this field and being a couples and family therapist is shifting the way I work to look at the participants and to find ways to observe as yet unobserved phenomena. Because my primary modus operandi in a therapeutic situation is to move people towards resolution states expediently I was aware that I often only saw such couples in moments of crisis and/or confusion. Even though I have been in the sex and gender diverse community myself for forty years, I still often did not get to see the analytic workings and psychodynamics of such couples operating in private. As my grandmother always said, "What you see on the street is not always what happens in the home."

For this project, choosing the first person singular narrative allowed the trans persons to tell their own story, which had always proved very revealing in our previous works, so both my co-editor Katrina Fox and I decided that it would be the most suitable way to go forward. When people memoir they often reveal more to the page then they ever would to the questions of a social scientist and a sort of hypnotic automatic writing takes over.

Questions that are posed by a researcher may intentionally be open but circumstances and expectations often produced highly filtered information; and even with the purest of intentions that can give rise to a sort of binary yes-no observation. In other words, I wanted to remove myself and Katrina as obstacles to the process of disclosure by those trans people revealing often deeply sensitive and private information about themselves and their love lives.

This, I can confidently say, has been produced in this book. It's what we might call the Swiss clock effect in that, through the stories, we are able to see many of the inner workings of the writer's mind. Such narratives often become reflective, self-analytical, and more revealing than any interviews could disclose. The results, I confess, have been surprising even to me. What I expected to find by reading the stories once they came in were strong patterns and themes that might run through the collective successful relationships. Or was I just hoping for a universal formula to sail the ships of trans people's love lives through the calm seas and storms of life?

As the reader can tell, what is revealed by this collection of stories is something quite different. The strongest theme that emerged is that there are few themes and that each relationship seems to have evolved or been designed, consciously or unconsciously, according to circumstance. The often tenuous nature of the bodies of trans people seems to give rise to a form of genesis when it comes to relations that by necessity had to abandon many of the formulae operated in relationships by average people with more stable body images.

Certainly trans people many have the desire and impetus to become involved romantically with others but in order to get to that point they have to negotiate an uncharted physical terrain of what goes where, when, and how. Added to that is the social complexities of frequently being in no man's land in a black and white world of male and female stereotyped gender presentations. Thirdly, having worked out all those complications, or at least the best ways of coping with them, the trans person has to deal with the oppressive intransigence and belligerence of laws that may preclude many trans people from legal relationship protection before the law.

In this book we have only heard from those trans people who, by design or circumstances, find themselves interacting with others in a romantic, loving, and sexual way. There are, however, many or in fact a vast sea of trans and intersex people who, through fear of rejection, never venture into the waters of love. They may have little confidence in their physical selves, poor self-images, and low expectations that anyone could ever find them attractive. Some trans people are so damaged by what is for them the trauma of being trans that they retreat into a world of seclusion, isolation, self-imposed ostracization, and post-traumatic mental illness.

The terrible prejudice, harassment, verbal, emotional, and physical violence that many trans people experience can scar them so deeply that they lose all basic trust in other human beings. Levels of trust that may be the very starting point for the ordinary person in the street may seem unreachably iconoclastic to a person who is constantly harassed in public simply for the way they look.

What is more to consider is the damage done to many trans people by overbearing and over-controlling clinicians all over the world who sift and sort them; depriving them of the human dignity to decide their own fate. After forty years of observing my peers in the international gender community, I have seen many people who have never recovered from the trauma of having their transition controlled by overzealous clinicians, who took away these people's very sense of ego. With very low self-confidence left after transition, they often entered into destructive relationships, turned to substance abuse, or ended up committing suicide. They do not number in the hundreds, but in the thousands.

The average sex and gender variance clinician is not aware of this because they do not frequent the ghettos, brothels, and prisons where these people often end up. Neither do many of the nice middle-class trans people who protect themselves with wealth know the extent of this worldwide holocaust of our trans community, because again, they too often stay in their safe zones.

Recently I sat talking at a major conference on sexology with a very well-known clinician and they asked what my area of interest was. I told them I was giving a paper on sex and gender variance with the use of the word "transgender" and one on autogynophelia/androphelia. When I told them, they exclaimed with horror that they had worked with "those transsexual people" as a placement after medical school and it nearly drove them nuts. "Those people are just too much work" I was told, and it never occurred to the clinician that I might be one of those dreadful people.

I cannot tell you, the therapist, how you should do therapy with trans couples because the mold is not made of stone. We as therapists use a mélange of techniques and skills from our accumulated kitbags, some of which come from our primary schools of therapy, others of which we steal like magpies from our endless attendances at workshops or even ideas we collect from books like these. What is important to remember is how creative and inventive people can be, particularly people who have needed to negotiate uncharted territories of body transmogrification.

If, like me and my partner Katrina, you have the utmost admiration for the inventiveness of the people who told us their stories of love in this book; you may concede to the fact that as therapists we are not the core motivators in couples therapy of any kind. With all kinds of couples counseling I do, however, establish certain basic rules:

1. I am not a referee.
2. I am not a judge.
3. I am not responsible for the success or failure of your couples therapy.
4. If you don't want to be here, leave.
5. My job is to simply to check in your coats, while you turn up as people in a relationship to work out and do the dance of resolution, solution, and propagation of respect.
6. I will be here offering you pointers and the rest is up to you.

I personally do not believe in the romantic notion that love will find a way. Relationships between any people require the basic pragmatics of rules of the road so that people have indicators and signposts by which to negotiate their worlds. Those indicators in medium to long-term relationship need to be known to all within that relationship so that safe boundaries can be established and negotiated without transgression leading to disputes and abuse, intentional or unintentional.

In short-term relationships the boundaries are far fewer and those involved are working in much shorter timeframes. Relationships for trans people are often built on short timelines since they can be quite unsure of their futures because many societies often do not afford them the stable protection of the law. This is similar to the pressures experienced by refugees, immigrants, and oppressed ethnic groups who have been unable to secure full citizenship and rights in their communities.

Even when trans people enter into longer, more stable relationships they can still experience major fears of rejection at some future date when partners get bored of living with the realities that their trans partners face each day. Those who have been in long relationships before transition may have greater ties to previous loved ones but also can experience greater incidences of rejection when revealing their trans ideation. Partners can perceive the transition as a great threat to their own identities and they can go into an identity crisis themselves as they have to reassess their own self-images. Those partners may experience feelings of betrayal, being deceived, or abandoned.

Some partners in those circumstances cope very well and become great adversaries of the trans person and may even continue platonic or even romantic relationships. In order for this to happen the partner needs to be very accepting and flexible; and the sort of person who is not bogged down by social constraint, overly religious dogma, or afraid of prejudice.

Romantic relationships for those who transition or cross-identify early in life pose a different set of questions and challenges. To reveal or not to reveal one's trans status is often the central key issue. For those who pass in society it can be very tedious and boring having to continually answer questions that they have answered a thousand times about their own identities that they see as no one else's business. There is also the fear the potential partner may reject them automatically before they get to know them, which can happen.

In an ideal world being trans might not matter, but we do not live in an ideal world. Trans people need to pick their moments to reveal or not and that will only come with experience of living in the new identity. I have known people who do not reveal at all, even to their partners and I respect their right to privacy. This situation can, however, sometimes be a bomb waiting to go off. Unexpected revelations can lead to the other person being angry that the trans person has not told them the information before. I have previously called this "living the secret" and it can be very stressful.

For the therapist, one of the most important issues in working with trans people is supporting and ego-strengthening in order to prevent self-denigration and low self-image. People are generally attracted to people who have positive images of themselves, even when that person is, or should I say, *particularly* when that person is trans. There are many people who are publicly trans, either purposefully through the way they present themselves or because their physiology and behavior identifies them as trans, who manage to have quite wonderful relationships. These people generally have good self-images and they have learned to be positive about their whole identity.

What we have not heard in this book is the stories of those people who fall in love and then go on to create families after transition which is becoming more common as laws change and technology produces such opportunities. In vitro fertilization (IVF) treatment for biological female partners of trans men and adoption for trans women has been very successful in many cases. Surrogacy has also helped some couples. In some cases there are people who have saved their eggs or sperm from before transition in order to contribute towards making children after transition.

The basic instinct to breed can be as strong in trans people as it can be in any type of person in society. Family therapists would be wise to encourage flexibility in the formation of family groups and instill in their clients openness if possible so that every family member can be accepted on their own terms as themselves. Parents of all kinds eventually learn that as you sow—so shall you reap—and love is never enough. Trans parents need to teach their children total acceptance of a wide range of human beings. Unfortunately, I have seen cases of families where the trans parents have become involved with religious extremism, and when the truth came out that they were trans, their children rejected them.

Therapists would do well to foster a sense of trans pride in their clients, couples, and families. Whether that pride is private or public is irrelevant provided it is operating as part of sustainable, positively-constructed ego and even superego. Anything less is denial and transference of transphobia on the therapist's part.

Therapists need to see sex and gender variance as a positive journey of self-discovery, and not just as a tortured path of self-destruction. The unhealthy obsession that to be sex and gender variant is a form of extreme psychopathology begs the question of whether the patient or the doctor should be wearing the white coat.

So what did I get as a therapist from this collection of trans people in love stories? To be honest, I got a sense of those relationships being organic. That is that the relationships seemed to fertilize themselves with a series of inventive dynamics that were born out of the need for the relationship to exist.

People, no matter who they are, seem to need to have relationships with other human beings. The interaction that takes place is undoubtedly food for the soul but also fulfills a physical need for human contact and love, which contributes toward homeostasis and growth.

We, the editors, are profoundly grateful to the contributors for trusting us enough to put forward their stories, but more than that, we are in awe of those contributors as human beings. I thank them not for teaching me more of what to do in therapy but for reminding me of the need for therapists to do less and allow the clients themselves to work out the healthy dynamics of their own relationships within a respectful environment.